The Conquest Of
PAIN

The Conquest Of
PAIN

Samuel Mines

GROSSET & DUNLAP
Publishers
New York

Author's Note: None of the medical or psychological procedures in this book should be undertaken except under the direction of a physician.

To Susan—wife, companion, bulwark

ACKNOWLEDGMENTS

A book of this kind would have been impossible to compile without the generous help accorded me by some of the country's most eminent doctors, whose help I gratefully acknowledge. In a very real sense these chapters are their personal chronicles, for they deal with and tell, largely in their own words, of the original research and discovery in the field of pain control that are broadening our vnderstanding of this ancient mystery.

In particular, I wish to express my debt to Dr. John J. Bonica, Director of the Pain Clinic at Seattle, to Dr. Richard G. Black, Co-ordinator of the Pain Clinic, who guided the many interviews there and who subsequently reviewed the manuscript, and to Dr. Benjamin L. Crue of the City of Hope National Medical Center at Duarte, California, who early read the greater part of the book and whose interest and encouragement were of particular and timely value.

Thanks go to many members of the Seattle Pain Clinic, including Dr. C. Richard Chapman, Dr. Wilbert E. Fordyce, Dr. Lawrence M. Halpern, Dr. Roy S. Fowler, Jr., Dr. Herbert S. Ripley, and Dr. Robert G. Parker.

Others who gave time and expert guidance include Dr. Richard A. Sternbach of the University of California, Dr. John W. C. Fox of Downstate Medical Center, Dr. Niels B. Jorgensen of Loma Linda University, and Dr. Jess Hayden, Jr., of the University of Iowa.

CONTENTS

Introduction

This book is about one of the most important concerns of mankind, a factor that has influenced the course of history. Certainly, there is evidence that man has been afflicted with this evil since his beginnings, for, as the records of every race are examined, one finds testimonials to the omnipresence of pain: on Babylonian clay tablets and papyri written in the days of the pyramid builders; in Persian leather documents; in inscriptions from Mycenae; in parchment scrolls from Troy. Down through the ages, in every civilization, in every culture, are found prayers, exorcisms, and incantations which bear testimony to the dominance of pain. "Were we to imagine ourselves," wrote the French surgeon Louis Dartigues, "suspended in timeless space over an abyss out of which the sounds of revolving earth rose to our ears, we would hear naught but an elemental roar of pain uttered as with one voice by suffering mankind."

While acute symptomatic pain serves the useful purpose of warning the individual that there is something wrong and acts as a practical diagnostic aid for the physician, in its chronic pathologic form pain is a malefic force which imposes severe emotional and physical stresses on the patient and his family. As Milton so eloquently stated in *Paradise Lost* (Book VI, ll. 462–64):

> *Pain is perfect miserie, the worst*
> *Of evils, and excessive, overturnes*
> *All patience.*

Chronic pain is the most frequent cause of disability and thus constitutes a major national and world health and economic problem. Although accurate statistics are not available, data from a variety of sources suggest that chronic pain states cost the American people over $25 billion annually. Costs include those of hospital, medical, and other health services, loss of work productivity, compensation payments, and litigation.

Even more important is the cost in terms of human suffering. It is a distressing fact that, in this age of marvelous scientific and technologic advances which permit us to send people to the moon, there are still hundreds of thousands, indeed, millions of suffering patients who are not getting the relief they deserve. Many of these patients are exposed to a high risk of complications from improper therapy, including narcotic addiction, or are subjected to multiple, often useless, and at times mutilating operations. A significant number give up medical care and consult quacks who not only deplete the patients' financial resources, but often do harm; some patients with severe, intractable pain become so desperate as to commit suicide.

Despite the importance of chronic pain, the amount of research in this field has been relatively small. The problem has never been approached as a major disease state—which is what chronic pain actually represents. Consequently, many gaps exist in our knowledge about the mechanism of chronic pain and other information essential to proper therapy of such syndromes. Moreover, because there is no systematic and organized teaching program for medical students and physicians which defines the proper management of these patients, the knowledge that is available is not properly applied. Another important factor is the trend toward specialization; each specialist, whether in research or health services, views pain in a very narrow tubular fashion.

Fortunately, during the past few years several changes have taken place which hold out the promise of eventual solution of this serious health problem. For one thing, there has been an impressive surge of interest among basic scientists in the study of the mechanisms of chronic pain syndromes; they have begun collaborating with clinical investigators and practitioners to solve some of the major problems. The field of pain research and theory, which had stagnated for almost a century, has recently been reborn—full of new controversy and renewed fascination. The simpleminded answers of the past are being critically examined and new questions are constantly being raised that challenge the investigator and point the way to new approaches in the control of pain. Furthermore, important advances in research and theory are being translated into effective clinical techniques. An important advance has been the activation of multidisciplinary pain "clinics"; these are composed of basic scientists and a variety of clinicians who collaborate in research, teaching, and patient care (as described in Chapter 7). Two recent developments are the founding of the International Association for the Study of Pain and the creation of the journal *Pain*. Both of these should prove effective in improving communication, encouraging greater research efforts, and speeding up the process of the application of new knowledge to the care of patients with chronic pain.

I am confident that this book will make a significant contribution toward improving the care of patients with chronic pain. Mr. Mines has done an admirable job of evaluating, distilling, and interpreting a vast amount of scientific information and presenting it in a lucid and easily readable manner. The book will appeal to the general reader and should be extremely useful for the victim of chronic pain, his family, relatives, and friends; it will help them understand the nature of pain and the physical, emotional, and cultural factors which contribute to this important medical problem. A valuable aspect of this book is the detailed discussion of both the advantages and the disadvantages of the most frequently used forms of treatment; it also evaluates the latest advances and therapeutic strategies in the field of pain research. Although the various procedures discussed in this book are useful when they are properly applied, patients and their families should be cautioned against expectations of complete relief of pain in every instance. The last chapter deserves special mention; it provides extremely helpful guidelines for the patient with chronic pain (and his family) on what to do and what not to do.

Practicing physicians as well as other health professionals should also find this book interesting and informative. The rather casual, unscientific style should prove a refreshing change from the typically rigid, organized, and often ponderous format of medical articles and textbooks. The book should prove especially useful to practitioners who have not had ample opportunities to gain experience in the management of chronic pain or to become acquainted with the various therapeutic modalities discussed.

Finally, it is hoped that this book will help the American people to better appreciate the importance of chronic pain as a national health problem and prompt the multipronged attack essential to the solution of this problem—greater research efforts, expanded clinical facilities, better teaching programs, and optimal patient care. These programs are best carried out in pain centers: multi-disciplinary facilities which provide the requisite environment for study, teaching, and service. To develop such centers, it will be necessary for the federal government, through the appropriate legislative bodies and health agencies, to provide adequate financial support and other resources essential to the success of these programs. As a consequence of these efforts, we may some day (hopefully very soon) learn much more about the complex nature of man's most vexing perennial problem—chronic pain. We will then be able to effectively relieve suffering humanity, which, in the final analysis, is the primary responsibility and the crowning achievement of every medical scientist and clinician.

JOHN J. BONICA, M.D.
Department of Anesthesiology
    and Anesthesia Research Center
University of Washington
Seattle, Washington

Chapter 1

THE NEW APPROACH
TO PAIN

*Although acute symptomatic pain serves a very useful purpose, in its
chronic pathologic form pain is a very malefic force which imposes
emotional, physical, and economic stresses on the patient, on his family,
and on society, and often taxes the diagnostic acumen and
therapeutic skill of physicians.*

JOHN J. BONICA, M.D.°

Man is born in pain, suffers pain through the crises of his life, and
unless he is exceedingly lucky, too often dies in pain.

For most of us, pain is inescapable, whether it be a trip to the
dentist, the drawn-out agonies of arthritis, low-back pain, migraine headaches, or a variety of crippling neuralgias.

Who has not awakened in the middle of the night to stabbing
pain and the quick rush of fear that follows? Yet the lancing pain
of emergency may be less serious than the chronic pain which
lays strangling hold, drains and devitalizes, distorts the personality, and even destroys the will to live.

Chronic pain is our most serious disabling disease. Its cost in

° Professor and Chairman, Department of Anesthesiology and Anesthesia
Research Center; Director, Pain Clinic, University Hospital, University of
Washington School of Medicine, Seattle, Washington.

human suffering is incalculable. Its cost in medical expense dollars has been estimated at $25 billion a year.

The average doctor does not even think of pain as a specific entity, but only as part of another problem, a symptom. We have learned better. There is pain which exists of and for itself.

As a result, a new specialty is emerging in medical practice: the therapy of pain. It is a specialty not practiced on an individual basis, like cardiology or obstetrics, but rather in a team approach, a multidisciplinary effort that brings together the skills of a number of medical specialists in a combined attack upon a condition whose underlying causes may be very obscure.

Nonorganic Pain. New research suggests something different about pain, particularly chronic pain. It undercuts the common conception that pain is no more than a symptom of something else, a warning signal of something wrong somewhere.

Frequently enough this is true. And in such cases, diagnosing and treating the underlying pathology should, and may, automatically dispose of the pain. In such cases, acute symptomatic pain has served the purpose of sounding a useful warning.

But thousands of people suffer from chronic, disabling pain with no discoverable pathology to account for it. In other cases the pathology is cured, but the pain doesn't go away. These are the cases, and they are legion, where the pain has taken on a malevolent life and become a disease in itself. It presents to the physician the problem of dealing with pain as an entity, divorced from organic malfunctions.

Not many physicians are prepared for this. There has been too little attention given to the study of chronic pain, in or out of medical school. There is, in all probability, an assumption everyone makes that the physician's responsibility is to diagnose and cure the illness or injury, with its accepted premise that pain has been the symptom. This in spite of the fact that chronic pain is a condition afflicting so many thousands of unfortunates.

The unpleasant fact is that we simply do not know very much about the mechanisms of pain. It isn't something you can see, or find upon dissection. There is even a growing distrust of the original assumption—that the primary purpose of pain is to sound a warning.

There are plenty of examples of pain which serves no useful

purpose: trigeminal neuralgia which causes excruciating pain in the side of the face; migraine; low-back pains; phantom pain—the pain that amputees feel in a limb they no longer possess. There are pains of psychogenic origin with no detectable pathology.

A case might be made that these are all warnings of a sort— perhaps of a disturbed emotional state, but if so, the pain is more likely to aggravate the disturbed state than to alleviate it.

Organic Pain. It must be acknowledged that pain, especially in the early stages, can be a clear signal of something organically wrong. In such cases it does perform the useful function of sending the sufferer to his doctor. In these cases there may be no great pain problem.

For example: The patient arrives at the doctor's office with a pain in his abdomen. It has moved to the right lower quadrant, he has vomited, and he feels quite ill. The doctor finds tenderness over the area called McBurney's point, takes a blood sample, and observes that the white cell count is way up. The diagnosis is appendicitis. The patient goes to the hospital and the surgeon removes his appendix, and after an appropriate healing interval, he is free of pain.

The surgeon cured his pain by removing the underlying pathology. No one specifically treated the pain, which was his original complaint. And the doctors were perfectly right; they knew the pain would go away when the diseased appendix came out.

Pain: A Disease. But there are a lot of people who do not fall into this easily diagnosed category. They hurt, and they continue to hurt in spite of anything the doctor can do, and the doctor does not know why. And pain that is intractable and prolonged outlives any usefulness it might have had as a warning and itself becomes a menace to health and life.

Pain is a menace when it forces people to risk narcotic addiction or to undergo ill-advised operations that may be multiple, useless, and mutilating.

Dr. John J. Bonica affirms that patients have come into the pain clinic at University Hospital in Seattle who have had as many as forty-two operations for low-back pain, with no improvement. Nerves have been cut, vertebrae fused, but the pain continued.

The record sharply contradicts the assumption that if you cut the telephone lines, the messages of pain are interrupted. Too frequently this is not true—the pain may continue.

Says Dr. Richard Chapman* "We can give a subarachnoid block (spinal anesthesia) to people, and I've seen this over and over again; they're numb from the nipple line down, and they still have pain."

Chronic pain is destructive when it leads patients to medical charlatans, forces them to spend their resources in a futile hunt for relief, or even drives them in desperation to suicide.

The recognition of chronic pain as a disease, and a disease of major proportions, came slowly, as the result of an accumulation of clinical data from many directions. A focal point was the publication, in 1953, of Dr. Bonica's massive volume, *The Management of Pain*,[1] a classic work in its field. It helped stir a handful of physicians and psychologists into a new perspective on mankind's ancient adversary, and the inadequate forces still available to deal with it.

Since the publication of this book, more than twenty years ago, progress has been made. A new concept, the pain clinic, has come into being. The prototype, and now probably the largest and best organized, was begun in 1961 by Dr. Bonica and Dr. Lowell E. White, Jr., a neurosurgeon, at University Hospital in Seattle, part of the University of Washington Medical School. Other pain clinics have been formed at other hospitals both here and abroad. What some of them have discovered about the nature and treatment of pain, and what hope they hold out for banishing pain, is the subject of this book.

There has been no attempt to cover all the pain clinics, or all the doctors working in this field, a task which would be beyond the scope of this work. The book is based on discussions with many of the best doctors in the country and is generally representative of the work now going on in a new and rapidly changing field.

* C. Richard Chapman, Ph.D., Professor, Departments of Anesthesiology and Psychology, and Anesthesia Research Center, University of Washington School of Medicine and College of Arts and Sciences, Seattle, Washington.
[1] Lea & Febiger, Philadelphia, Pennsylvania.

Chapter 2

THE NATURE OF PAIN

*Most people have been brought up in our culture to think of
pain as a sensation in the form of input, like vision, or hearing.
Pain is not a sensation.*

BENJAMIN L. CRUE, M.D. °

Any serious investigation promptly turns up two irritating discoveries:

1. Things are not what they seem.
2. They are always more complicated than you expected.

Take both of them as axioms regarding pain. To the person
who is hurting, theory may seem maddeningly academic, but it
is the essence of the problem.

Let's say you have burned your finger, and it hurts. It had been
assumed in a general way that an injury damages tissue, and that
this affects special nerve endings in the skin called nociceptors
which react to injury or pain. From these receptors the message
of tissue damage travels up along the telephone lines to the
spinal cord and thence into a pain center in the brain where it is
recognized as pain. Right? Wrong.

° Chairman, Division of Clinical Neurology; Director, Department of
Neurosurgery, City of Hope National Medical Center, Duarte, California.

Pain Without Anguish. Consider the Indian fakir who plays hop-scotch barefoot on a bed of fiery coals, with no visible evidence of anguish. What messages travel along his nerve pathways from foot to brain, and how does he interpret them? As pain, or something else? Is there a qualitative difference between what he feels and what you feel when you burn your finger?

Among a number of American Indian tribes, torture for captured enemy warriors was a noble institution. The captive himself would have been grievously insulted not to be put to torture. And while his enemies were artistically carving him up, or slowly roasting him, he would sneer at their efforts and describe in detail how much better he could do the job if their positions were reversed.

A film shown to doctors in the pain clinic at Seattle featured a headache treatment by a witch doctor in Uganda. The patient, who suffered from chronic headaches, had the choice of going to a Western-style hospital or to his local witch doctor and chose the witch doctor. The operating room was a clearing in the forest. The witch doctor, who was a kind of folk medicine specialist, brought out some rusty knives and other utensils, shaved the victim's head, then cut the scalp down the center and once across, peeled all the skin back, and with a crude drill bored holes in the skull—apparently to let the pain out. He then put back the flaps of skin and the patient went home with his head taped. At no time did he show any sign of pain, nor did he have any kind of anesthesia.

In all three cases, the question, naturally, is: were all these people superhumanly stoic about pain, or did they actually feel something different from pain as we think of pain?

And a further question, which ties the two together: how much of this is related to cultural background and conditioning? Can these factors affect one's perception of pain?

In our own culture, we seem to take it for granted that the Latin types are more voluble, emotional, and expressive than Anglo-Saxons. We somehow expect an Englishman or Irishman to be more stiff-upper-lip about pain and less verbal than an Italian or Frenchman. Army experience indicates that this is so. It proves nothing about the courage of any of them, nor does it tell us anything about the way they feel pain. It merely indicates the cultural format in which they express themselves.

Awareness of Pain. Conditioning is one element. Distraction or concentration is another. Here's a football player who goes through a tough game and later, in the shower, a teammate says, "What's that bump on your shoulder?" He discovers that he has a broken collarbone. Once he knows it, it starts to hurt. Until then, he didn't feel it and didn't know he had it.

How many times have you been absorbed in some task, to find later that you'd cut yourself and never felt it at the time? How many children come running to show mother a bleeding cut or scrape acquired in fast play about which they show only curiosity, appearing to feel no pain?

Apparently, concentration or distraction plays a large part in the perception of pain, just as does cultural conditioning. Both situations have this element in common: they illuminate the puzzling fact that even where a direct physiological injury is involved, pain is not necessarily a simple cause-and-effect phenomenon. In both cases there are extenuating circumstances which complicate things.

The plot thickens considerably when we get into areas where there is no injury or disease, and not even detectable stimuli to cause pain, yet pain occurs.

KINDS OF PAIN

Pain can be acute or dull, transient or chronic. The differences are important.

Acute transient pain is usually the result of infection, injury, or internal disease. If the cause is properly diagnosed and treated or removed, the pain is usually eliminated.

But suppose the cause cannot be removed, or even discovered, and the pain continues over a long enough period to be classed as chronic? This becomes much more troublesome and difficult to handle. Dr. Bonica groups chronic pains into three main categories.

Referred Pain. The first group he calls "persistent peripheral noxious stimulations," coming from pain signals generated by long-term disease conditions of many kinds—arthritis, ulcer, herniated disk—even cancer. The pain resulting from these conditions, and the side effects such as muscle spasm, tenderness, and so on, may not even be near the actual site of the problem. This is referred pain.

The reflex responses to this kind of pain and to malfunction caused by injury or disease tend to perpetuate themselves, fed by a variety of stimuli surrounding or resulting from the condition; this sets up a kind of vicious circle in which the pain disturbs bodily functions and causes more pain.

Pain and trauma may bring on sufficient emotional stress to provoke muscle spasms, digestive disturbances, and constriction of blood vessels, with diminished flow of blood to vital organs, all of which set in motion a new cycle of problems.

Neural Pain. A second group of chronic pain conditions are those involving the neuraxis, or brain and spinal cord. These include various forms of neuralgia and a few serious diseases of the spine or brain.

Learned Pain. The third group are the "operant mechanisms," which means simply learned pain behavior. There are certain bitter rewards for being sick. The patient's behavior in signaling pain has brought increased attention, sympathy, and notice from those around him. It has excused him from tasks which may have been distasteful, lifted responsibility, and brought him, perhaps, better treatment than he normally expected. There is a chance, under these circumstances, that he may develop a pattern of chronic pain behavior which outlasts the original pathology.

This is neither conscious nor malevolent. The patient continues to suffer, and he may be totally unaware that he is part of the pain problem. It can be deadly serious.

A young woman came to a pain clinic with a condition of chronic pain that had lasted for years, had seriously incapacitated her, and had so restructured her life as to dictate her activities, her friendships, and her total existence. She told the doctor who examined her that she was desperate, that she had been unable to get relief anywhere.

The doctor was young and enthusiastic about his work. Upon completing his examination he was happy to tell her that he believed he could help her. Even where the cause of the pain is unknown, he told her, there are simple procedures like nerve blocks which can totally relieve the pain. He guaranteed, he said, that if she returned the next day, he would remove her pain. The young woman thanked him, went home, and committed suicide.

"That was a bad lesson," the doctor said. "And I learned it the hard way. She didn't really want to have her pain removed. She had structured her whole life around it. She couldn't handle it, she wouldn't know how to face the day that she woke up without pain. What would she do—what would she now be expected to do? How could she manage? She just couldn't deal with it. That lesson I have never forgotten."

Chronic pain does not become more tolerable with time. On the contrary, pain appears to sensitize the system so that suffering becomes worse the longer it continues.

"Protracted pain," says Dr. Bonica, "whether moderate or severe, produces physical and mental depletions which vary widely from one person to another, and may be evidence of basic personality differences. The presence of general debility, malnutrition, fatigue, anxiety, or mental turmoil further decreases the tolerance of the individual to pain.

"As a result, the pain is more severe and more difficult to treat. Lack of sleep is particularly important in this respect. The patient with chronic pain exhibits a gradual but complete alteration in his attitude toward his environment. Consequently he loses interest in all other activities, and the pain becomes a consuming problem which completely dominates his life."

Chapter 3

HOW WE FEEL PAIN

*Neurosurgeons thought that if you cut the telephone wires you
don't get any pain messages, but in fact you do get messages.*
                                    RICHARD G. BLACK, M.D.°

Charlie Brown of the "Peanuts" comic strip says, "Pain is when
it hurts," and unfortunately there isn't much in the way of a
better explanation than this, although a lot more words can be
used.

Nerve Fibers and Pain. Toward the end of the last century, a
German anatomist named Waldeyer propounded the neuron doctrine, which defined the basic unit of the nervous system as a
neuron, or nerve cell. The cell consisted of a nucleus, a long axon
or nerve fiber with branching dendrites from the nucleus and
bare nerve endings from the lower end of the axon. These bare
nerve endings were seen as sensitive receptors to pick up stimuli
which were transmitted along the axon as a kind of built-in telephone line to pass the stimulus along.

   The chain of nerves did not form a solid line. There were tiny

   ° Assistant Professor, Department of Anesthesiology and Anesthesia Research Center; Coordinator, Pain Clinic, University of Washington School
of Medicine, Seattle, Washington.

gaps between the branching nerve ends of one cell and the next, like spark plug gaps, which were called synapses. As a charge built up in one cell, it could fire across the synapse to the next, the impulse being an electrochemical reaction quickly damped by an enzyme so that the process was kept under control.

Nerve fibers were classified in three groups:

Class A fibers are large fibers enclosed in a fatty sheath called myelin. They have a high excitability and conduct impulses relatively fast, from 5 to 100 meters a second.

Class B fibers are medium-sized myelinated fibers with a lower excitability than Class A fibers, and a conduction rate of 3 to 14 meters a second.

Class C fibers are thin, unmyelinated or only slightly so, with a conduction rate of 0.5 to 2 meters a second.

C fibers are considered to be mainly conductors of pain, although A-delta fibers and B fibers have been found to show some response to pain. Primarily, however, A fibers were considered responsive to touch, pressure, and temperature, while B fibers had more to do with visceral and other internal sensations.

Experiment showed that touch was conducted rapidly while pain traveled along a slower impulse, corresponding to the A and C nerve fibers. One study showed that asphyxia blocked the faster impulses first and predictably abolished the sense of touch before pain was affected. Cocaine blocked the slower impulses first and, again predictably, screened out pain before touch. There seemed, therefore, to be empirical support for the belief that the large fibers carried the sensation of touch and the small fibers carried pain. In fact, the relationship turned out to be fairly loose, since the larger fibers also carry pain to some extent.

But the general classification of neurons was a start on the way to a theory of pain. Since nerve cells differed widely in the type of bare endings, or receptor organs, it was inevitable that there was an attempt to classify these as specific for each type of sensation.

Specific Receptors Theory. The doctrine of specific nerve endings was first suggested by Sir Charles Bell, a physiologist of Edinburgh, in 1811, and later expanded by Johannes Müller. If you stimulate one kind of receptor, Müller said, you get one kind of sensation, and no other. Thus, in the skin there are specific receptors for cold, heat, pain, and touch—each one different and specific.

The experimental work seemed to bear him out. Investigators located specific points on the human skin where any kind of stimulation produced a single sensation. For example, you could touch an ice cube to a heat receptor and get the sensation of heat, with another receptor the ice cube would give only a sense of pressure, and so on. This was the theory of specificity—specific receptors. It did not go unchallenged.

Pattern Theory. It was, in fact, opposed to a much earlier concept that pain was merely the extreme of any sensation. Really intense stimulation of the skin with any of the other three sensations—touch, heat, or cold—would produce the fourth, pain, if it were only intense enough. This concept had been proposed by Erasmus Darwin in 1793, and was essentially the basis for what later came to be called the pattern theory, in opposition to the theory of specificity.

In 1858 specificity got a boost when a German physiologist named Schiff demonstrated that cutting through the gray matter of the spinal cord abolished pain below the incision, yet did not affect the sense of touch. And cutting the white matter of the cord reversed the process, eliminating the sense of touch, but not pain.

Schiff's work was picked up by others in the nineteenth century, notably Goldscheider and von Frey. Goldscheider agreed that there were specific "pain points" in the skin, where only pain sensations were evoked, but pointed out that they were bunched so closely together and required such varying degrees of stimulation in order to react that he could not agree there was a special type of receptor for pain and pain alone, or that pain was therefore a distinctly separate sensation.

Von Frey insisted that there were individual, specific receptors for pain, with different ones for touch, each producing its own type of sensation only. And this was the beginning of a long and sometimes bitter controversy down through the years.[1]

[1] The theory of specificity was further strengthened by E. D. Adrian, who demonstrated that stimulating the nerve endings of touch fibers, up to

THE MELZACK-WALL GATE THEORY

In November 1965, a paper appeared in *Science* [2] titled "Pain Mechanisms: A New Theory," written by Dr. Ronald Melzack and Dr. Patrick D. Wall.[*] The authors agreed in some respects,

the very limit of their ability to conduct, still did not produce the sensation of pain.

S. W. Ranson and his collaborators identified the pain neurons as the small, myelinated and unmyelinated fibers found in mixed nerve roots. Waterston, experimenting on himself by slicing layers from his skin, found that the epidermis was where touch is felt and the corium was the area of superficial pain.

The controversy seesawed back and forth. The English school of Weddell and Sinclair picked up Goldscheider's findings and elaborated them into the pattern theory. Their work convinced them that all fiber endings, whatever their morphological differences, were basically alike and it was the intensity of the stimulus that determined whether it was pain or another sensation that was felt.

W. K. Livingston, supporting the pattern theory, argued that there were so many different kinds of nerve endings that the likelihood of their all falling into just four types, each limited to producing one of the four sensations, was very small. It might be, he said, that under normal conditions, activating one type of nerve ending might result in a certain sensation—touch or pain. But this did not mean it would always be so under all circumstances. The sensation could be modified by any number of changing conditions—the type of stimulus, the condition of the receptors at the moment, or a host of influences in the body which might affect the pickup and transmission along the telephone lines all the way from the skin to the brain. Pain, Livingston said, is a central perception coming from many impulses which are synthesized as a total sensation greater than the sum of its parts. It is, therefore, a new entity.

Nevertheless the specificity theory was generally accepted and taught in medical schools. Some diehards held out against it. W. H. Erb, in Germany in the last quarter of the nineteenth century, continued to teach that pain was the result of intensity of stimulus.

Goldscheider amassed considerable clinical evidence that there were no such things as pure pain receptors. Livingston and Haugen found that in the cornea of the eye, and in the teeth, which are supposed to be supplied only with pain receptors, touch can be felt. And in cases of surgery for trigeminal neuralgia, where the root of the trigeminal nerve is cut to relieve intense facial pain, touch sensation in the cornea continues, even though it is equipped only with so-called pain endings.

[2] Vol. 150, No. 3689, pp. 971-79.

[*] Ronald Melzack, Ph.D., Professor of Psychology, McGill University, Montreal, Quebec. Patrick D. Wall, M.A., D.M., Professor of Anatomy; Director, Cerebral Functions Research Group, University College, London, England.

and disagreed in others, with both the specificity and pattern theories. They proposed instead the now famous "gate control" theory.

Briefly and oversimplified, the theory postulated the existence of a gating mechanism which could swing shut to selectively block out pain. This hypothetical gate was considered to be located in the gray matter of the spinal cord, in the material called the *substantia gelatinosa,* which is part of the "dorsal horn" where the peripheral fibers come in and are switched to the central transmission fibers or T cells, on their way to the brain.

The gating mechanism is supposed to work somewhat in this fashion. If a stimulus is applied to the skin, both large and small fibers respond. As we have seen, the large fibers are supposed to carry the sensation of touch, the small fibers the sensation of pain. As the intensity of the stimulus increases, it floods the gate, which is very sensitive to the critical balance between large and small fibers, as they continue firing. If the large fibers are overloaded, there is feedback through the short neurons of the *substantia gelatinosa,* the gate swings shut and stops the pain signals from coming through. The mechanism of the gate is modulated by impulses from the brain area, in other words, the responses to the pain signals.

In real-life situations it might work this way: you bang your elbow going through a doorway and pain knifes up your arm. Your reaction is to rub the injured spot. The rubbing loads the large fibers, the gate closes, and the messages of pain from the small fibers are cut off. The elbow starts to feel better.

You jab your finger with a pin. You put the finger in your mouth and load the large fiber receptors with the sensation of warmth. Or you rub the spot, with the same result.

In their discussion, Melzack and Wall considered the deficiencies of other pain theories. With regard to the theory of specificity, they noted that cutting a nerve did not always abolish pain below the cut as it theoretically should; they noted that gentle touch can sometimes trigger excruciating pain and that sometimes pain occurs without any stimulus at all—at least any external stimulus. They even noted that a gentle rubbing, repeated pinpricks, or application of warmth to the skin can, surprisingly, trigger a delayed reaction of pain after half a minute or so.

Looking at the pattern theory, they rejected an explanation of pain as a simple relationship between the severity of the stimulus and the pain response. They noted the psychological factors which affect sensory input. They cited Professor H. K. Beecher's observation on the Anzio beachhead [3] that American soldiers wounded in the invasion often did not feel pain, presumably because they were so relieved to find themselves still alive and now effectively out of any further combat.

In one of Pavlov's famous experiments with dogs, the animals were subjected to electric shock or other pain stimuli, which was immediately followed by an offering of food. In time the dogs responded to the pain as a signal that food was to follow, and thenceforth failed to show any sign of pain whatever.

As Melzack and Wall point out: "If these dogs felt pain sensation, then it must have been nonpainful pain, or the dogs were out to fool Pavlov and simply refused to reveal that they were feeling pain. Both possibilities, of course, are absurd." The conclusion was that a stimulus strong enough to produce pain can be deflected or modified into a signal of something else, in this case of eating behavior.

The pattern theory failed to cover the facts, they felt, because it ignored the fact that there is definite physiological specialization among neurons. It would therefore be more reasonable to assume that the specialized nature of each receptor-fiber unit affected the response to a stimulus on the skin.

The Melzack-Wall gate theory stirred up a great deal of interest, and reawakened the old debate, with new elements added. Dr. Benjamin Crue, Chairman of the Division of Clinical Neurology of the City of Hope National Medical Center, disagrees in part with the Melzack-Wall theory. "The gate theory is a simplification, and it's a beautiful job, and it deserves all the credit it gets."

But he considers it wrong on three counts. First, it set out to bring about a marriage between pattern and specificity theory, and didn't. "They do not understand, because none of us does, how pain is transduced at the peripheral endings, so they begin their diagram with a large fiber and a small fiber coming in. Well, we all know there are large fibers and small fibers, and the small fibers somehow have more to do with the patient's feeling pain.

[3] H. K. Beecher, *Measurement of Subjective Responses*, Oxford University Press, New York, 1959.

But that doesn't mean you can go back to the skin and say, 'Well, the pain stimuli are there.'"

The term "nociceptor," Dr. Crue believes, has caused confusion because neurophysiologists do not equate nociceptors with pain endings, but clinicians do. "Clinicians naturally think of nociceptors as pain endings, as is implied in the derivation of the word itself. However, in my opinion, there is no such thing. The physiologist realizes that the term nociceptor merely means a high threshold mechanoreceptor or a thermoreceptor.

"When you stop and think about it, there are no such things as pain stimuli. There are only stimuli that are painful by analogy. And this isn't a semantic play on words to get out of a difficult situation; it's a really different change in concept.

"When you classify senses you've got to look at the forces on the intact skin that are sufficient to bring about what we call a stimulus, that bring about changes which can then be interpreted in the central nervous system as 'it hurts.'

"If pain is only felt in the presence of tissue damage, and pain is per se a chemical stimulus, then we in neurosurgery and neurophysiology are wrong. But we have been going on the assumption that you can feel pain without tissue damage.

"If this is true, the only thing that the surface, the intact cutaneum, can tell you is that there has been either mechanical deformation or thermal change. That's the *only* thing the skin can do.

"Now you can carry it to the degree where touch becomes pressure and then becomes painful, and whether you use a pointed pin or something not sharp, there is still no such thing as a pain stimulus but only mechanical deformation to the point that it's painful.

"This is so basic that you can't approach the Melzack-Wall theory without realizing that they've left out the whole outside-of-the-fence story. You can't ignore the argument between specificity and pattern theory, you've got to come to grips with it and settle it. Personally, I think that Weddell and Sinclair and the English school were correct, and the pattern theory or some form of it, is right.

"We've gone back and tried to reclassify the primary senses. The idea of five senses is so ingrained that when you talk about the sixth sense to the layman you're talking about clairvoyance and telepathy and parapsychology and Rhine's experiments at Duke—or the new program on television. The sixth sense is anything that doesn't fit in with those five. And in medicine we're still going along using those same five senses.

"Now this goes back to Aristotle; this is over 2,000 years old. We think it's time for a change in our classification of the basic senses. And we want to reclassify the basic senses as the forces, the energy sources, in nature that can cause an adequate stimulus. And that means there's no such thing as pain." [4]

His main objection to the gate theory deals with the transmission cells. "The T cells that transmit the impulses onward and upward to consciousness, where it is interpreted as pain, Melzack and Wall envision as lying there waiting for something to happen. The theory suggests that this balance of input between the large and small fibers may or may not fire the T cells. Well, that's wrong. It can't work that way and you can get two conditions that can't be explained by the theory.

"One is when you fire an abneuralgic (distant from the central nervous system) pain in trigeminal neuralgia (intense pain in the side of the face). You can precipitate this by touching the lip and the patient feels pain. You send in a nice burst of touch information over the large fibers and the patient interprets this as pain. The gate theory doesn't explain this.

[4] Dr. Crue continues: "You have an adequate stimulus, whether it's pressure, or too much heat, or too much cold. But it causes the right pattern when it goes in, and certainly there's sensory modulation in the region of the dorsal horn, and Melzack and Wall deserve a lot of credit for bringing this to our attention.

"Whether it works exactly the way they describe is a question; there are a lot of good neurophysiologists who say that it doesn't. The thing we find fault with at the gate itself is that Ron Melzack and Pat Wall state that this gating is done by pre-synaptic inhibition, built up by feedback from post-synaptic activity. It's really a change in the polarization of the primary afferent. And our point is that if you can do this to the point that you can control whether or not the *substantia gelatinosa* lets the impulse through, depending upon whether it's a large or small fiber, it's very easy for us to believe that this pre-synaptic inhibition carries up until it reaches threshold and fires, and you get antidromic (going the wrong way) impulses in the dorsal roots.

"This has been Dr. Carregal's and my interest for the last seventeen years. This isn't just a gating, there's a blocking with extinction by dorsal root activity." E. J. A. Carregal, M.D., is affiliated with the Departments of Neurosurgery and Clinical Neurological Research at the City of Hope National Medical Center, Duarte, California.

"The second is phantom limb (pain apparently coming from an amputated member). The neurophysiologists have talked about perturbations in this neuroma stump (new growth largely nerve cells and fibers), but the clinicians have known for years that you can take those neuromas out and it usually doesn't stop the pain. You've got to explain pain syndromes in the absence of input.

"We think the T cells are capable of independent action. They are command cells. And under pathological conditions they are hypersensitive. Usually because they've had a change in their input. We've known about this for years. It's called de-afferentiation hypersensitivity. And when you have these T cells whose input has been cut down, they are capable of firing independently."

In short, Dr. Crue believes that *all* pain—stick a pin in a normal, healthy individual and it is the same phenomenon—is uncontrolled repetitive firing in the T cells.

Dr. Crue cheerfully admits he holds a minority opinion.

"If we're right about uncontrolled repetitive discharge in these neuron networks in layer five in the cord, it is so incredibly complex that we can't go to the blackboard and wrap up a schematization of how this works. There are so many inputs from below and potentiation from above that you just can't simplify it nicely."

Dr. Kenneth L. Casey[*] studied and collaborated with Dr. Melzak on a number of papers. He recently wrote the following in the *American Scientist:* [5]

"There is currently much debate about the gate control hypothesis. . . . The complexity of synaptic arrangements there obscures any decisive anatomical evidence for or against the gate hypothesis."

Four years after his original article appeared in *Science,* Dr. Melzack wrote an editorial for *Anesthesiology.*[6] The early model of the gate theory, he said, was probably wrong in several details, but more important was the possibility that by the very controversy it stirred up, it would encourage new laboratory

[*] Associate Professor of Physiology, University of Michigan Medical School, Ann Arbor, Michigan.
[5] "Pain: A Current View of Neural Mechanisms," Vol. 61, No. 2, March/April 1973, pp. 194-200.
[6] "Evolution of Pain Theories," Vol. 31, No. 3, September 1969, pp. 203-4.

work to test out its hypothesis. New facts are already available "which go beyond the gate control theory; they, together with other recent data, already begin to indicate the need of a new theory of pain."

This is the process, Dr. Melzack said, by which science progresses. A theory stimulates new work which leads to a new theory. "Herein lies the power of the scientific process; it promotes the growth of concepts and ideas that have an organic continuity in a way that resembles life itself. We must learn to give up old and cherished ideas, painful as the process may be, because this is the only way scientific progress can occur."

Chapter 4

THE PSYCHOLOGY OF PAIN

It used to be pretty easy to label somebody a hypochondriac when you couldn't find a physical explanation for pain, when it didn't fit into your nice diagnostic categories. But I'm seeing an awful lot of people who hurt, who are pretty healthy, resilient, effective people.
And to take away their hurt you don't have to give them psychotherapy, and you don't have to change their whole lives. You don't have to look for a purpose or a good explanation for it—you just change the pain behavior.

DR. ROY S. FOWLER, JR.[*]

We have seen that despite areas of controversy among our experts, there is substantial agreement on our two original basic premises.

1. Pain is not what it seems, a simple cause-and-effect mechanism, but is largely subjective.
2. Pain is very complicated, with so many psychological factors that those most concerned with it admit frankly they still do not know what it is.

[*] Associate Professor of Psychology, Department of Rehabilitation Medicine, University of Washington Medical School, Seattle, Washington.

As one commentator put it, "Physical pain is not a simple fact of nervous impulses traveling over a nerve at a predetermined gait. It is the resultant of the conflict between the stimulus and the individual." [1]

"Pain is a classification imposed on something we feel," says Dr. Richard Chapman. "It's a categorization we carry out on some kind of input to the brain from the outside. The information that comes to the brain is largely nonspecific, it's a barrage of neural impulses. When this information carries any kind of unusual intensity it's classified as pain. It doesn't matter necessarily what sensory modality you're dealing with—too bright a light, too loud a sound, too strong a taste, or too intense a cutaneous stimulation. These things are all classified as pain. The readiness of a patient to call something that he feels 'painful' may depend on his personality or the social situation he is in.

"Socially we tend to reserve the word 'pain' for things that are related to tissue damage, toxicity, and the like, so there's a correlation of tissue damage with pain. But there's no necessary cause-and-effect relationship. Pain is said to exist when the individual complains of it. You can't cut into the body, into the brain, or into the skin, and find pain, nor can you do an EEG (electroencephalogram or brain wave recording) and see the pain. Pain is an altogether private experience."

The concept that pain does not require tissue damage is well recognized. In 1938 F. M. R. Walshe wrote, "In psychogenic pain, none of these anatomical mechanisms of physiological processes is involved, and the symptoms so named have no sensory quality to which the term 'pain' can rightly be applied. They are not primary sensations but complex states of mind, emotionally toned ideas which would be more fittingly described as 'anguish,' 'grief,' 'distress,' or 'anxiety.' The subject of psychogenic pain should rather be said to have a fixed idea or obsession about pain, or alternatively to be using the word pain figuratively because he cannot more adequately describe the distress of mind from which he suffers. Thus stated, the difference between physiogenic pain and psychogenic pain should be clear." [2]

It is clear that pain cannot be separated from emotion, and

[1] R. Leriche, *The Surgery of Pain*, Bailliers, Tindall & Cox, London, 1939.
[2] "Psychogenic Pain," *British Encyclopedia of Medical Practice*, 12 Vols., London, Butterworth & Co., 1936-9.

that emotion plays a major role in the perception of pain, increasing it in some cases and blocking it in others. A group of war prisoners who were subjected to pain punishment or torture varied considerably in their reactions to pain. Some said they survived by learning to "turn off the pain." [3]

If we can accept even partly the gate control theory, we can recognize in it the inhibitory action of the brain on the input of pain sensations through the closing of the gate.

In a new paper, the collaborative work of Dr. Melzack and Dr. Chapman,[4] they discuss the therapeutic implications of the gate control hypothesis:

1. Pain can be controlled in some situations by increasing large fiber output, such as that initiated by massage or tactile stimulation.
2. Pain can be modified by maximizing central control factors by means of specific training, e.g., behavioral conditioning, or by using suggestion and distraction.

The importance of the psychological factor can be seen where pain situations that make one individual a tragic invalid are shrugged off by another as relatively minor. What are the factors that affect or alter the experience of pain?

"Perception" is all-important. How do we perceive pain? One element in perception is attention. When you give your full attention to something, be it an object, a person, an emotion, or an event, you block out other things competing for notice and you focus all your faculties on this one subject. That process can increase the pain or be used to relieve it.

Suggestion is one method of affecting attention in acute pain, although its effects are unpredictable. One experiment studied was the use of white noise (a generalized sound like the rushing of wind) as an auditory stimulation to distract a patient's attention from dental drilling. White noise coupled with suggestion brought relief from pain, but either one alone did not.

The conclusion reached was that suggestion was more important than the white noise. Dentists with strong personalities, who were able to make convincing suggestions that it was going to

[3] S. Wolf and H. S. Ripley, "Reactions Among Allied Prisoners of War Subjected to Three Years of Imprisonment and Torture by the Japanese," *American Journal of Psychiatry*, Vol. 104, 1947, pp. 180ff.
[4] "Psychologic Aspects of Pain," *Postgraduate Medicine*, Vol. 53, No. 6, May 1973, pp. 69-75.

work, had more success than those who had their own doubts about it, or who attempted no suggestion but merely gave the patients the headphones for listening, without some kind of pre-conditioning. The patients, too, differed widely in their suggestibility.

Anxiety can produce feelings of fear which lead to increased activity of the autonomic nervous system—rapid heartbeat, changes in breathing, sweating, and so on—which can rise rapidly from distress to actual pain.

Skeletal muscle tension, says Dr. Herbert S. Ripley,[*] is a common cause of pain. A vicious cycle is set up in which the pain further increases the muscle tension which again intensifies the pain. Anxiety, anger, or depression can affect the contractions of the smooth muscles of the gastrointestinal tract and produce abdominal pain. Emotional reactions can affect the tension of the chest muscles and produce pain and tightness, which may be mistaken for a disturbance of the heart.

Depression can reinforce pain and may be the cause of pain by itself. The chronic pain patient is frequently a depressed personality—introspective, self-punishing, accident-prone, or hypochondriacal.

Another condition is classed as "hysterical pain," traditionally explained in psychoanalytic theory as an attempt to cope with buried conflicts in the personality. But a simpler explanation [5] is that hysterical behavior is a cry for help, and the patient is adopting the extremisms of hysteria in a desperate effort to reach someone who otherwise will not, or cannot, be reached.

If this theory is correct, say Melzack and Chapman, hysterical pain should not be considered as a symptom of undiagnosed pathology, either organic or psychiatric, and it must be treated with different means than the conventional medical therapy.

The pain reaction can be altered by conditioning. If an individual has been encouraged, or even permitted, to associate a strong emotional reaction with pain in early life, even minor pains later on may trigger strong emotion and severe suffering.

[*] Professor and Chairman, Department of Psychiatry, University of Washington School of Medicine, Psychiatrist-in-Chief, University Hospital, Seattle, Washington.

[5] See T. Szasz, *The Myth of Mental Illness*, Harper & Row, Inc., New York, 1961.

Variation of pain behavior among patients is very great, and in some it does seem excessive for the amount of observable tissue damage.

Social factors are also of importance. We have touched upon the real, if dubious, rewards of illness or pain. Melzack and Chapman make the further point that individuals who are invalided by chronic pain are rarely well adjusted or successful. This seems harsh, and undoubtedly there are exceptions, but as a generality it appears to be an unpleasant fact that many such people build for themselves a small universe enclosing their pain, and a behavior pattern that victimizes family, friends, and even their physicians.

How does this happen? Melzack and Chapman say, "Life is a stream of ongoing behavior. The direction behavior takes is determined by environment. When behavior is followed by an environmental event that is in some sense rewarding or satisfying, the probability that the behavior will be repeated is increased."

The patient is not the only victim of this kind of conditioning. "A physician who is reasonably successful in his personal and professional life has little reason to modify his behavior patterns. The patient, however, may be lonely, frustrated, alienated, and generally dissatisfied with life. When an accident or illness generates simple pain behavior, the patient may experience more rewards for being in pain than he obtained in his normal routine."

Dr. Wilbert E. Fordyce[*] describes the housewife who discovers that her back pain brings new attention from a husband who was otherwise rather indifferent to her. This attention and sudden solicitude and helpfulness are very attractive, even though they are contingent upon her continuing to hurt. "Hurting leads to help and attention, non-hurting does not." [6] There is no conscious malevolence involved, perhaps not even a conscious ulterior motive. Therefore, if the pain behavior continues, there is only the fateful consequence that her pain behavior has been reinforced by a pattern of reward.

Man is a social creature, needing identity and relationships to

[*] Professor of Psychology, Department of Rehabilitation Medicine and the Pain Clinic, University of Washington School of Medicine, Seattle, Washington.

[6] "An Operant Conditioning Method for Managing Chronic Pain," *Postgraduate Medicine*, Vol. 53, No. 6, May 1973, pp. 123-128.

prevent a sense of isolation and alienation.[7] If a career fails to provide this sense of social identity, the role of chronic invalid may offer an alternative.

The role of invalid provides in a tragic way a rich life of attention and activity. It offers visits to or from physicians, relatives, and friends, much sympathy, challenging projects in the way of proposed surgery or rehabilitation therapy—in short, an identity which heretofore may have been lacking. Those who become "career patients" are often cooperative, even submissive. They visit their doctors faithfully, take what is prescribed for them, but somehow do not stop hurting. They become expert in discussing their symptoms; like patients in analysis they learn a pseudo-language of medical terminology. All of which gives them the identity they seek, structured around the central keystone of pain.

Obviously these are questionable rewards, and the end result is self-destructive. A life-style of invalidism undermines whatever is left of health and character. In some cases, multiple surgeries, as Dr. Bonica has affirmed, can be all too common, are often useless, damaging, and mutilating.

For the chronic pain patient there is also the possibility of drug abuse. The search for an effective pain killer may lead the patient to collect an arsenal of prescriptions, often from different physicians, and to swallow these drugs in varying combinations with no idea of the general effects, the side effects, or the interaction possible between drugs.

Dr. Lawrence M. Halpern* tells of one patient who was taking hundreds of dollars worth of medication a week, prescribed for her by seven different physicians, none of whom knew anything about the others. "She was taking one drug every four hours, another every four hours, another every six hours, another every three hours, and then the first drug again at bedtime. She was taking that stuff faithfully and she had no idea the drugs were making her ill when she came in.

"With others you prescribe a drug four times a day and suddenly find they're taking a hundred pills a week. And they're

[7] See Eric Fromm, *Escape from Freedom,* Farrar, Straus, New York, 1941.

* Associate Professor, Department of Pharmacology and the Pain Clinic, University of Washington School of Medicine, Seattle, Washington.

doing that by themselves, and that's a whole different ball game in terms of how you self-medicate a patient, or how you allow them to have drugs, and what they're doing with the medication."

In what has been said so far, there is no intent to put all chronic pain sufferers in the class of professional pain patients adopting a pattern of pain behavior because it offers more in the way of reward than their normal life does. Melzack and Chapman agree that it must be assumed all pain is real, inasmuch as it is real to the sufferer. And pain behavior is a signal to the doctor that he is to provide help. What he also needs to determine is whether this signal indicates emotional stress rather than disease, and how this affects his treatment.

There are people with genuine emotional distress and with real reason to hurt, in the absence of tissue damage. With intelligent help their pain can be diminished or banished, and they are glad to see it go.

"I think," says Dr. Roy Fowler, "the public pretty well accepts the fact that ours is an uptight society, and if you're uptight it's not unreasonable that you'd hurt. But you know, there's really not a whole lot of good data.

"It does appear that different people respond in different ways to the same kind of stressful stimulus. Some people will respond with a stomach problem, some people will respond with a cardiac arrhythmia (irregular heartbeat), some people will respond with an increase in muscle tension, others will respond with a change in their galvanic skin resistance. There are a number of different ways in which different people respond. You can present the same stimulus but they'll respond differently. But there aren't good data to support the conclusion that all these things called tension pain are, in fact, related to excess muscle tension."

Pain resulting from major tissue damage may require heroic measures in the way of drugs or surgery. But psychological factors can be used to reduce pain, sometimes from unbearable levels, at least to bearable levels. A planned program using relaxants, sedatives, and tranquilizers often makes pain seem less important, and we will hear more of this from Dr. Halpern in another chapter. Suggestions, placebos, biofeedback, acupuncture, hypnosis, and electrical gadgets—all have been used effectively, as has a major tool, nerve block, to break up pain patterns or stop pain, and we will discuss these individually.

Where there is little or no tissue damage, say Melzack and Chapman, and psychological factors may be involved, it behooves the physician to gain perspective on the causes, and the environmental and personality factors that keep it alive.

Many family physicians are finding themselves forced to provide psychological counseling in lieu of traditional therapy. In these cases the doctor can try to help the patient develop some insight into his problem, to suggest alternative behavior and solutions, and to encourage the patient to single out those people, or those environmental factors, which support his pain behavior by offering rewards.

In short, conclude Melzack and Chapman, pain is very complex. It may be a warning of disease, a bid for attention or sympathy, a signal of unhappiness or depression, or merely a characteristic way of reacting to other people. Whatever it is, it presents a puzzle to the physician who is called upon to do something about it.

How can he determine if pain is emotionally induced? Short of putting the patient through the hospital's endless gauntlet of tests to eliminate any organic condition, Dr. Ripley suggests a quicker method sometimes used by psychiatrists. This is to administer intravenously sodium Amytal, or sodium Pentothal. Either drug promotes relaxation. If the pain is due to emotional causes, it nearly always disappears. If not, it is probably due to causes other than emotional. This effect of sodium Amytal lasts only an hour or so, which makes it of limited use therapeutically, but it is a good diagnostic tool.

Dr. Ripley cites the case history of a woman patient invalided by severe leg pains. "She'd been a very active woman whose chief hobby was golf, and she'd had to give it up. The source of her pain was not clear. We gave her intravenous sodium Amytal, her pain disappeared, and she started talking about how she had gotten upset and sort of given up after her mother had moved in with her. Her mother demanded that she be a loyal, attentive daughter, and her demands were unceasing. She was getting no satisfaction out of life, yet she felt she couldn't ask her mother to leave. She had to do her duty, her mother had been good to her for years, and so on. She brought out all these conflicts.

"These were then discussed with her and she was able to get them in perspective. Mind you, the conflict doesn't automatically disappear, but with insight the patient can handle it differently.

"She had to learn that insight isn't enough, it has to be put into practice. She had to learn to say to her mother, 'I'm not going to stay home with you all the time. I have my own life to lead. I am going to devote a certain amount of attention to you, and I'm going to be supportive, but I have to have some life of my own.'

"It was difficult and painful for her to assert herself. She did not like to hurt her mother, but once it was done, she found they got along better because her mother gained more respect for her. And instead of her mother going to pieces, as she feared, and being more accusatory, her mother said, 'Well, I guess you're right. I've been selfish and demanding.' It worked out to a better relationship without her mother becoming alienated."

Pain is associated with punishment, but there are circumstances under which it can become a source of satisfaction or even pleasure. Sadistic parents enjoy inflicting physical punishment on their children, but there are children who enjoy being spanked. There are instances too numerous to describe of both sadism and masochism in sexual relations.

Freud believed that both were included in the sex drive and that one was likely to become dominant. Children brought up in rigidly restrictive homes, and punished for indulging in various pleasures, may become pain dependent. Says Dr. Herbert F. Ripley, "The individual, by punishing himself in advance, may thus attain license to gratify his forbidden desires, and the anticipation of pleasure overrules the deterrent action of pain. Thereby pain becomes a paradoxical stimulus for pleasure, enhanced in its value by the unique esthetic effect of contrast." [8]

Dr. Ripley has done some experimental work on the importance of suggestion in the experience of pain. One experiment is meant to induce pain by means of a headband fitted to a volunteer, which is tightened to the point of a fairly high level of pain. The headband is then removed, the subject is hypnotized, and the suggestion is made that he will go through the experience of having the headband put on again and tightened. The headband is not put on, but the subject develops pain again just as though the band were being tightened, and reports that the pain is so excruciating that he cannot stand it.

[8] "The Psychologic Basis of Pain," Chapter 4 of *The Management of Pain* by Dr. John J. Bonica, Lea & Febiger, Philadelphia, Pennsylvania, 1953, pp. 143-154.

Part of this psychological approach to pain, at least where it clearly involves tension, is to promote relaxation by whatever means appear effective, from sodium Amytal to hypnotism. Post-hypnotic suggestions, says Dr. Ripley, are not uniformly effective, but help many people, even cancer patients, for whom they serve to reduce the quantity of narcotics needed to keep them comfortable.

Relaxation is of benefit in migraine, or in smooth muscle spasm, even though the musculature is not under voluntary control. The relaxation of skeletal and other voluntary muscles contributes to the easing of tension and relaxing of muscles under control of the autonomic system, with a likely easing of pain.

Dr. Chapman stresses the point that in his work at the University of Washington he is a research psychologist, not a clinical psychologist.

"I see things a little differently from an M.D. I haven't been 'acculturated'—trained in medical school for X number of years that this is how you think of patients and interpret what they say. I look at chronic pain as behavior. Here's a patient sitting in a room waiting for me, pre-set to demonstrate pain behavior, and he's probably been emitting pain behavior at home, at work, and so on. I'm going to go in there and interact with that patient's habitual behavior patterns, and I'm wondering what things determine this individual's actions, habits, and perceptions.

"I'm interested in how people make themselves sick and how they make themselves well. And I'm beginning to think that a great deal of what medicine contends with is exactly that. Of course, one can't explain all problems in this way, but I suspect that a substantial proportion of patients fall into this category.

"People seek help because they are sick, and in some cases they've either made themselves sick foolishly, or they've done it intentionally at some subconscious level. A great deal of what we call cure, even if it follows neurosurgical intervention, occurs because the patient is now ready to change his life and get rid of what he was doing before.

"I happened to stumble upon a fellow in the hospital cafeteria about a year and a half ago, who was a gastroenterologist. He told me that about 80 percent of what he sees in his internal medicine practice is what you would call psychosomatic—has no explanation, there's nothing organically wrong. All kinds of expensive tests are carried out on the patient and they don't reveal anything. Eighty percent!

"It seems to me that we should ask, 'Why is this going on?' I would guess that a great number of people are stressed because of social or personal conflicts. When I say that, I mean emotional double-bind situations, interpersonal stresses, business stresses, economic stresses, a sense of inadequacy, failure to reach one's goals—all those things. They all hang in together.

"If you've got a wife or child who is acting badly toward you or toward society, that's a stress too. These things add up. When a person is stressed, the autonomic nervous system reacts. You know what intense stress feels like if you step off a curb when you didn't see a car. When he hits his brakes and you turn and look at him, you notice that suddenly your heart is racing and you're short of breath, and there's sweat on your forehead.

"Well, this kind of reaction, although more subtle, goes on with long-term stresses also, though the conscious brain can't detect it. You may look at your body and say, 'I feel fine,' but your body is not in its natural state of balance. The sympathetic and para-sympathetic parts of the autonomic nervous system are not pulling together as they should be. And after a period of time, structural changes occur. The most obvious of these probably is the peptic ulcer, but there are many others.

"One might hypothesize that in the patient under emotional stress there is too much activation of the sympathetic nervous system, or too little, a great deal of the time. Chronic backaches and muscle aches might reflect too little sympathetic activation. Sweating and hyperfunction of any sort could be too much activation. If this be so, the endocrine system and the autonomic nervous system are major contributors to pain problems.

"The body is quite capable of putting itself back together again, but the conscious mind may be repeatedly interpreting things as threat and continually working up the defense mechanisms of the body. Such defensive reactions are adaptive on a short-term basis, but destructive when continued for too long a time.

"Most of our psychotherapy is exactly this kind of thing—controlling the autonomic nervous system, as in one approach to phobia, where you teach the patient the Jacobson method of relaxation. The patient lies down, clenches his fists, relaxes, clenches his arms and relaxes, tightens his thighs and relaxes—it's a training that takes several sessions until the patient is completely relaxed and feels like he's floating. You can then condition him to accept the experience of things he's normally frightened of."

Dr. Chapman, who has experimented with acupuncture, believes this may be one of the effects of the needle, that it can bring about an effect of relaxation very quickly. It may tend to reduce physiological stress reactions.

"I think there is at least this physiological impact to it. But you ask, what's a stress? Now the old Chinese physician, the classical one, like you never see any more, might see a patient and the patient would show X number of problems. And he would say, 'I can treat you. I can cure this. But I won't do it unless you change the way you're living, because the problem will just come back again. It isn't worth doing unless you change the way you're living.'"

Not many Western doctors do this. If they see signs of stress they are more likely to prescribe a tranquilizer, which, of course, can be helpful for short-term relief. But the patient isn't usually compelled to consider how his habits affect his health.

"Depression in a patient reflects stress, and people are often depressed because they're angry. At Duke University we helped a severely depressed man using the Jacobson technique for relaxation and took him off tranquilizers eventually. This was a man who could never express his hostility or anger—at his boss, or family, or anyone. He was always a nice guy. He had a phobia about saying anything nasty to anybody, so we taught him to do this in fantasy while relaxed and eventually he could express himself by saying, 'I don't like it when you do that.'"

What this patient had to learn was a method of expressing his anger without appearing to be nasty, to do it in a civilized, even considerate fashion. He would need to be able to say to his daughter, for example, "I don't want you to play your stereo that loudly, it disturbs me," rather than to yell at her to shut the damned thing off.

This patient was one of a minority of people who do not subscribe to the commonly accepted idea that it is unhealthy to repress anger and that people are better off for letting it all out. For him it was more distressing to let it out than to hold it in.

He was more disturbed by the thought of hurting someone else, and this was part of his problem. He had to change the way he was behaving in order to get better.

"Some patients need to learn to say things in an adult way. You know—'I've got a problem with you, friend, and this is my problem. Now, how are we going to work this out?' It's a way of getting things done. If you feel a frustration, solve the problem by removing the obstacle, or adjusting your goals, not just smoldering in anger."

Since he is not a clinician, Dr. Chapman does not see patients on a regular basis. But he sees enough of them to have begun to think in terms of techniques for helping them, based on what he is learning about stress.

"I'm becoming intrigued with psychosomatic concepts in medicine. I think these ideas can account for what is going on in acupuncture therapy and a lot of other things. There are many chronic pain patients who get better briefly with everything a physician does. Surgeries get them better, but the pain comes back. Acupuncture gets them better, but it still comes back. Psychotherapy gets them better, but the pain comes back. Drug X gets them better, but the pain still comes back. It comes back because of the way they live.

"We treated a woman with tic douloureux (trigeminal neuralgia) in this clinic with acupuncture and got dramatic relief a couple of times. Thereafter it was impossible to help her. Interestingly, this lady's pain is triggered by almost any loud noise, and do you know what one of her hobbies is? Bowling. Her husband gave her a bowling ball for Christmas, which tells one something about the marriage.

"The games some people play contribute to the deterioration of their health. To stop playing them is the hardest thing in the world, because that's how they meet their needs. But it's wasteful to treat anybody physiologically for problems that are just being generated by interpersonal stresses that don't have to be there.

"In some instances physicians treat people like we repair cars in the local garage. The car comes in and there's something wrong with the carburetor so the mechanic rebuilds it; puts it back together again, and the car runs. But a human being is a dynamic, ever-changing, critically balanced machine and sometimes you've got to look at the whole machine, not just fix the carburetor. It doesn't always work when you do the obvious mechanical thing."

Not surprisingly, the neurophysiologist, or neurosurgeon, looks at the problem a little differently.

"We haven't got the answer," says Dr. Crue. "Not in medicine or psychiatry or psychology for the 'chronic benign pain syndrome.' And while I'm interested in pain and what pain is, I'll have to admit quite frankly that I don't have any answers either. I think I know a little bit about the neurophysiology of pain, and understand what pain is, and can go a little bit beyond Melzack and Wall's gate theory. But when it comes to treating people, I end up giving aspirin because it helps most headaches. From an empirical, symptomatic standpoint, it works. And when we get to the ones that don't, we use Sternbach's multifaceted approach.[9] And there is no question but what, in this day and age, most of these people who come in, if you give them tender, loving care, and are a supportive father-figure or psychologist, give them antidepressants, tranquilizers, muscle relaxants, and work with them, then *most* patients can be helped. Even when there's underlying pathology.

"There is almost *always* underlying pathology. This idea of pain for secondary gain, or purely psychoanalytical pain—the right side of the patient's face hurts because her lover slapped her there as he left her in the cold night and walked off into the black darkness and never came back—this may happen—I'm not saying there can't be psychogenic pain, but that is an extreme rarity. In 99 plus percent of the functional pain problems we get, there's a reason why it's in the left face, or in the left shoulder instead of in the right. There's an old injury there—there's underlying pathology. *Almost always.* But it is being potentiated, exaggerated, consciously or subconsciously, and that is your chronic pain syndrome."

What is needed in treating chronic pain, in short, is what was derisively called shotgun medicine in the old days. Now it is called a multifaceted approach, and it is used because there are no miracle panaceas, like a magic analgesic.

"What we've got to do is to learn to use the best medication in the right dose at the right time for this patient with a particular syndrome. Along with good psychiatric care. And by using an

[9] See Chapter 11.

intelligent shotgun approach we can help most of these patients. But there are still a lot of failures."

And much can be done by diligently searching out and correcting any underlying pathology that can be found. People with headaches or facial pain may have dental problems, or they may not.

"There are those patients with a lot of functional facial pain and it's psychiatric and it's anxiety, but if you do correct the malocclusion and give them a decent bite, the syndrome goes away. You can correct, in some patients, the underlying pathology, even though it's minimal, and if at the same time you've got them on the right tranquilizer in the right dose, and you're following them along and give them psychological support, then at times you may succeed in relieving the pain.

"All of these things tie in together. And this is what a modern pain center has got to be. It's got to be multifaceted, you can no longer have a pain center where you sell one thing."

The modern pain clinic, typified by the one at University Hospital in Seattle, is just that.

"For proper management of the patient with chronic pain," says Dr. Bonica, "at least three requirements must be met. First, a detailed history must be obtained and a complete work-up done, including neurologic, psychologic, and sociologic evaluation.

"Second, the mechanism of the pain must be determined. We have found it helpful to classify chronic pain states as due to persistent peripheral noxious stimulation, chronic diseases of the neuraxis, or operant mechanisms.

"Third, treatment must be planned carefully, considering such factors as the patient's age, life expectancy, and obligations.

"Meeting these requirements is a time-consuming process, for which a multidisciplinary team approach is ideal. However, the physician who is willing and able to devote the necessary time to the problem can achieve good results." [10]

We shall have a look at the modern pain clinic shortly.

[10] "Fundamental Considerations of Chronic Pain Therapy," *Postgraduate Medicine*, Vol. 53, No. 6, May 1973, pp. 81-85.

Chapter 5

WITCH DOCTORS, SPIRITISTS, AND MYSTICS

The whole of early medicine was saddled with a rag-bag of preconceptions which we now regard as "unscientific," although as medical fashions change, and the interaction of mind and body are more closely studied, our appraisement grows less complaisant.

PENNETHORNE HUGHES [1]

Let's digress for a few minutes from the purely scientific to the spiritist or outright magical. There are two reasons for this digression.

One is historical. Witches and faith healers played an early important role in treating pain and disease, and are yet far from through. The second reason is that we need to consider the role of the mind and emotions in both disease and cure, and remember their very considerable contribution to both.

To primitive and medieval man, illness and pain were clear signs of possession by evil spirits, unfriendly gods, or demons. The believer's only recourse was to turn to his local sorcerer or witch doctor to exorcise the demon and remove the pain.

By the Middle Ages witchcraft was a flourishing profession,

[1] *Witchcraft*, Penguin Books, Baltimore, Md./N.Y., 1965.

albeit with a mixed reputation. There was a clear-cut distinction between such innocuous pursuits as herb medicine or faith healing, both reasonably respectable, and outright witchcraft, which was allied to the dark powers and to old Beelzebub himself.

There were, however, white witches, who used their powers for healing and helping, as well as the black witches who figured so prominently in the duckings and burnings which enlivened the scanty entertainment of the day.

Busily cooking up charms and spells, witches had a smattering of folklore pharmacology (mixed with a heavy dose of superstition regarding the efficacy of such ingredients as bats' tongues and dried toad) together with other arts which were called into use for brewing love potions, ensuring the fertility of wives, and curing cattle of bovine ailments. In like manner, the dark witches professed to casting spells which could make cows go dry, wives barren, cause headaches, lameness, abortion, and various other interesting ills.

They knew enough so that if the magic failed, they could administer a noxious herb to human or cow, and produce the desired effect. The biblical word for witch, as well as the Italian, translates to "poisoner," and in the Middle Ages they were frequently accused of poisoning wells, spreading plague, and selling poisons of various sorts to their customers.

As medicine outgrew its early dependence upon astrology and incantation, it began the long process of discrediting witchcraft. Yet witch doctors, faith healers, and voodoo priests knew something the modern physician has only recently rediscovered, the power of the mind. Saints and witches had one thing in common, an apparent immunity to pain.

Saints chanted hymns as they burned at the stake, raising their arms as a signal to the next victims that they felt no pain. The Essenes, a monastic brotherhood of Jews in Palestine, defied the most vicious Roman tortures. Muslim dervishes known as Sufi plunged knives through their flesh and smiled. The voodoo practitioners of the West Indies juggled red-hot pieces of iron, stirred boiling water with their hands, danced in fire, or ate broken glass without the slightest sign of discomfort.

Go back earlier and you find Egyptian priests practicing hypnosis, telepathy, and autosuggestion, with evidence that they could exert their powers at a distance, as voodoo experts are supposed to do in the West Indies and Africa. The Egyptians mastered a form of body control similar to that practiced by the Yogi today, a system of sublimating the body and detaching the consciousness. By breath control and concentration, they were able to create striking changes in the power and energy of the body and the conscious mind.

Witch doctors effected "cures" by magic, which is to say that folk medicine played a part and the superstitious beliefs of the subject did the rest.

The secrets, such as they are, of the witch doctors are still zealously guarded. Certainly, "spells" and the "evil eye" are straightforward examples of suggestion; there is strong doubt that a victim would be affected by a spell if he didn't know about it. There is plenty of evidence that once he did know about it, he would be strongly affected. A pin through the heart of a voodoo doll might very well kill the original of that doll, so long as he knew the pin was there. If he didn't know about it, the result would be much less likely.

There are many recorded trials of witches for these and similar crimes; a famous one in England goes back to the year 1324. Robert le Mareschal of Leicester denounced a male witch in Coventry, along with twenty-seven of the witch's clients. The charge was a plot to kill the King together with the Prior of Coventry and several others, for which the witch was to be paid twenty pounds and Robert le Mareschal fifteen pounds. They had made figures of each of the victims, and as a trial run they had made a figure of an innocent bystander named Richard de Sowe, and had thrust a pin through the head. De Sowe obligingly went out of his mind, and when a second pin was pushed through the heart of the doll, he died.

This convincing demonstration scared le Mareschal sufficiently so that he decided he wanted no part of the plot, turned state's evidence, and fingered the witch, who was arrested.

The curious thing always about these stories is that the great powers of the witch seem to fail once he or she is in jail. One would think he could easily influence his captors, or simply part the iron bars and walk out. But it doesn't seem to work that way. The witch of Coventry, like so many others, was executed without difficulty.

The idea of possession by demons was never alien to the theological doctrine of any age. Greece may have seen the dawn of the scientific age, but people believed in all kinds of spirits—bad and good. Socrates, for example, owed his wisdom to the guidance of good spirits, and it was only when they deserted him that he was offered a hemlock cocktail.

The early Christians limited demons to evil ones, attributing misfortune and suffering to the malicious attentions of these occult busybodies, who apparently had little else to do but haunt people.

Cures by faith, or the laying on of hands, has a long history. In the 18th century there lived in London a lower-class Irishman named Valentine Greatrakes. A humble man of no education, he was greatly surprised to have a dream in which he saw himself curing the sick by the laying on of hands. At first he dismissed the notion, but the dream was recurrent, and he began to suspect that someone was sending him a message. He decided to try this supposed power and, by good fortune, a subject was at hand, his wife, who had pains in her stomach. Greatrakes cured her, to his own astonishment, and quickly gained a reputation as a healer. His fame spread, and he was invited to work his miracle on the royal family. Playing it safe, the royal family called in the Bishop to supervise, and all turned out very well. The Bishop, impressed, observed Greatrakes' work for several more weeks and testified that Greatrakes was honest and of sound moral character.

Simply by his touch, said the Bishop, Greatrakes "drove the pains to the extremities of the limbs. Many times the effect was very rapid, and as if by magic. If the pains did not immediately give way, he repeated his rubbings and always drove them from the nobler parts to the less noble, and finally into the limbs."

Among the diseases the Bishop testified he saw Greatrakes cure were "dizziness, very bad diseases of the ears and eyes, old ulcers, goiter, epilepsy, glandular swellings, scirrhous indurations, and cancerous swellings."

What was important about Greatrakes is that he evidently influenced a Frenchman named Franz Mesmer who, across the Channel, was groping toward a therapy enlisting "animal magnetism" and hypnotism.

Mesmer was a physician who had abandoned conventional medicine for a theory that diseases consisted of foreign forces, by which he meant interplanetary forces, in the astrological sense, that were acting on the body. To cure a patient, it was necessary to purge the body fluids of these invading forces.

Mesmer believed in group therapy. He sat his patients around a huge wooden tub filled with "liquid matter." He connected them to an iron rod, the other end of which went into the tub. The patients joined hands and, with the addition of song or background music, diffused their magnetism into the tub, sending the foreign forces along with it. Patients were also individually mesmerized, or hypnotized, by oscillating a finger or wand in front of their eyes, a technique in use by some hypnotists for the same purpose today.

The Royal Medical Society of France jeered at Mesmer, the clergy branded his methods as witchcraft, but a lot of patients pronounced themselves cured of their ills, which is no surprise.

Mesmer's vogue passed, but what he had started was picked up and adapted to their own use by others, notably Emanuel Swedenborg of Sweden, who went into trances and talked directly with God, by which means he effected miraculous cures.

The most proficient operator of the eighteenth century was a faith healer named Joseph Balsamo, who gave himself the title of Count Cagliostro. He became famous throughout most of Europe, and was called the Divine Cagliostro. At the height of his career he treated five hundred people a day and was showered with wealth and honors.

Balsamo was an uneducated peasant born in Palermo, Italy. He found his chosen profession of confidence man quite early and, as a young man, was invited to leave town after being exposed as a fake medium who had cheated the local jeweler out of his savings.

He then accumulated a grubstake through another old device —using his wife Lorenza as the lure in the common blackmail setup. The wife lures a victim into the bedroom and the outraged husband appears. His wounded honor can only be salved by a handsome cash payment.

The couple next appeared in Russia, at the court of Catherine the Great. Balsamo had now become Count Cagliostro, the famous healer. Having boasted that he could cure anything, he was invited to cure a case of total baldness and when he was unable to produce hair, he was invited to leave Russia suddenly.

Communication being very slow in those days, the failure did not damage his credibility elsewhere. He and his wife appeared in Strasbourg with a retinue of servants, in an elegant carriage. He took the best accommodations at the best inn, while his servants spread the story that he was a sorcerer who possessed the fabled philosopher's stone that could change lead into gold and cure all ills.

The organization showed considerable imagination. One of his servants, asked how old the Count was, replied that he didn't really know, since he had been in the Count's employ only a few hundred years. He was, however, able to remember the exact day he was engaged because it happened in Rome the very day that Julius Caesar was assassinated.

Count Cagliostro entertained visitors with his personal recollections of the Trojan wars, repeated intimate conversations he had had with Helen of Troy, and asserted that Cleopatra was no great beauty in spite of her reputation.

Then came the pitch. He could cure all ills, but would treat only the poor, and for free. He would have nothing to do with the rich.

The lame, the halt, and the blind moved in. They converged upon Cagliostro in a flood. He made a sign on their foreheads, or touched a drop of elixir to their lips, and they threw away their crutches and walked. Pain vanished, limbs distorted by ancient agonies straightened themselves out.

The miracle was there for all the world to see. Now, attracted by the spreading clamor, Cardinal de Rohan arrived. He was rich and powerful, so presumably off-limits for one treating only the poor and downtrodden. But he was a holy man, and Cagliostro consented to see him. The Cardinal had an ailing relative. Would the Count be good enough to work his miracle?

Cagliostro graciously agreed. He laid on his magic touch and the sufferer was well within the week. The Cardinal was overwhelmed. He was also intrigued by the notion that Cagliostro could turn lead into gold. He suggested they leave Strasbourg and journey to Paris.

Cagliostro was ready to go. In fact, it was high time he left. Many of his cured patients had relapsed, and some had died. It was time to move.

In Paris he let himself be persuaded to heal the rich and to accept a fee. He sold a miracle chair which would cure the pains of rheumatism if the patient merely sat in it. He offered a powder that made women beautiful, and an elixir dipped from the Fountain of Youth, which turned back the ravages of time.

He took Paris by storm. Money poured into his pockets. Artists painted his picture, sculptors carved busts of him. He was so much the vogue that his picture adorned lockets and ladies' fans.

Then a fatal mistake. He became involved, apparently innocently, in a scandal with Cardinal de Rohan over a diamond necklace. De Rohan, in fact, was framed by the Comtesse de Lamotte, who got him to sign a voucher for a diamond necklace she said Marie Antoinette had asked him to purchase for her secretly. De Rohan, who was in love with the Queen, was glad to do it.

But the Queen knew nothing about the necklace. The Comtesse had invented the story and pocketed the necklace. When the bill came due, de Rohan was unable to pay. Marie Antoinette ordered the arrest of de Rohan, the Comtesse, and Cagliostro, who was known to be intimate with de Rohan.

The trial cleared Cagliostro of complicity, but his image was shattered. Paris no longer held him in awe. His cures failed to work. With his wife, he left Paris for Rome. There they were arrested for membership in a secret society, tried by the inquisitorial court, and sentenced to life imprisonment. The flight of the Divine Cagliostro was over.

Miracles come in all sizes and packages. David St. Clair, an American journalist who has spent much time in Brazil, has witnessed and gathered accounts of some incredible instances of miracle cures.[2]

Brazilian Spiritists banish pain and illness by sending magnetic rays from their fingertips into the "magnetic fluid" of the patient. We all have an aura, or fluid body, around our physical bodies, say the Spiritists, and this fluid can be unbalanced, just as our physical organs can be. The Spiritist can spot an unhealthy mind or body instantly by the color of the aura.

Health produces a blue-white aura, illness a gray one. There is a second aura which shows the state of mind and emotions. Blue is spiritual, orange indicates ambition, red violent passions, pink love, green treachery, gray depression, and so on.

[2] *Drum and Candle,* Doubleday & Co., Inc., Garden City, New York, 1971.

When the Spiritist lays hands on a patient, he is acting like a battery to send good electricity into the aura and "push out the particles that are in conflict with the others." No doubt Edison would have been intrigued to learn that there is "good" electricity and "bad" electricity. But disease, according to these spiritual healers, is no more than electrical particles that have gone haywire.

But the laying on of hands is small potatoes indeed compared with the exploits of an unlicensed Brazilian healer and surgeon named Arigó. This is a stage name; his real name is José Pedro de Freitas. Arigó means "country bumpkin," a name adopted in deference to his beginnings as a farm boy and his continued reputation as an unspoiled, simple son of the rural life.

The official version of Arigó's story is that he is possessed by the ghost of a German doctor named Fritz, who appeared to him in a dream and told him he would cure the sick and afflicted. Apparently Dr. Fritz really takes over, for when Arigó operates, the simple Brazilian farm boy disappears. He speaks in a heavy German accent and wields a scalpel like an obsessed surgeon. He undertakes any kind of surgery, slashing, cutting, and gouging with frightening speed. He removes tumors, cataracts, and cancers, and performs major abdominal surgery such as colostomies.

He operates without anesthetics of any kind, using a kitchen knife, a pair of nail scissors, and tweezers, which are stored without sterilization in a rusty tin can. He cuts and draws no blood, and heals wounds by simply drawing his finger over the incision. His reported exploits are fabulous.

A typical case was that of a teen-aged boy with one leg three inches shorter than the other. He also had a heart condition and was considered a poor risk for major surgery. According to the story, given wide credence in Brazil, Arigó put the boy on an army cot, took knife and meat saw, cut off the good leg, shortened it by three inches, put it together again, passed his hand over the wound, and the boy walked out with two good legs the same length. All this was done without anesthesia of any kind.

A Brazilian senator is reported to have come to Arigó with a lung tumor so advanced that doctors in both Rio and New York had declined to operate on him. They spent the evening together drinking, and just before he passed out, the senator had an illusion that Arigó disappeared, or turned into a little fat, bald man in the white jacket of a doctor. In a heavy German accent, the little man announced that he was going to take out the tumor.

When the senator awoke in the morning, he told Arigó his dream. Arigó scoffed at it, insisting he was a good Catholic and had no truck with ghost stories. He denied knowing anything about surgery and insisted they look at the bedsheets for signs of blood, and at the senator's back for an incision or scar. There was nothing.

The senator went home and to his doctor, where X-rays were taken of his lungs. "A beautiful job," said his doctor, "whoever did it. The tumor is completely gone, and they've even done an outstanding plastic job in eliminating the scar."

This is the stuff of legends, and there are dozens of similar stories about Arigó, who became so famous in Brazil that bus tours were run to his home. It is alleged that his operations have been filmed, showing him checking the bleeding by saying, "Let there be no blood, Lord."

The church became unhappy about Arigó, and the law has made numerous attempts to stop his unlicensed practice. Once he was arrested and sentenced to a prison term, but he was immediately pardoned by the president, then Juscelino Kubitschek, apparently to operate on one of the president's daughters.

It is also told that a medical team arrived from Berlin to observe Arigó and, during an operation, held a lengthy technical conversation with "Dr. Fritz" in perfect German. Dr. Fritz identified himself as a German surgeon who had been killed in World War I. He didn't work alone, Dr. Fritz said. He was helped by an equally deceased French opthalmologist named Dr. Gilbert Pierre, and a Japanese tumor specialist named Takahasi. They did have an anesthetist, the spirit of one Friar Fabiano de Cristo, who sterilized the instruments and administered an ethereal anesthesia by means of a mystical green light.

Dozens of witnesses, permitted near the operating table, have heard Dr. Fritz call out for "more green light," although since he is supposed to speak in German, it is curious that all these Brazilians understood him. They immediately got so much more green light that it spilled over into the first ring of spectators, who instantly passed out.

Apart from the stereotyped names of the long-dead medical team, there is no explanation of how an obscure German army surgeon had acquired such superhuman skills.

For example, St. Clair describes a session he personally witnessed, which tops the other stories. He was allowed into the operating room, an ordinary square, white-painted chamber, with a single window and a wooden bed on which was a straw mattress. A wooden door, laid over two carpenter's horses, was the operating table. About twenty people lined the walls, waiting for the healer.

Arigó came in, walked to the patients and looked closely at them. The first, a woman, he cut off when she tried to tell him her symptoms. He told her her trouble was in her spine, that she should stop drinking so much coffee, and wrote out prescriptions for drugs she was to take.

The next patient was a man with a tumor the size of a lime under the skin of his upper arm. Arigó took a knife, but did not cut. He merely rubbed the blade over the skin. The tissues parted without any bleeding and the tumor popped out. He took a piece of cotton, passed it over the wound, which instantly closed, and dismissed the patient. There remained no scar, no sign of any incision.

The next patient was a woman with a tumor in her back. It received the same treatment.

The final patient was a blind teen-aged boy. Arigó, or Dr. Fritz, helped him up onto the table and asked him if he was afraid. The boy said he was not. Dr. Fritz told him to relax.

What follows, St. Clair reported in all seriousness.

Arigó took a kitchen knife and thrust it straight into the boy's right eye. Brusquely he pried the eye out of the socket and held it in his hand. Next, taking a scalpel, he went back into the eye socket and dug away at something in the back. Then he put the eye back.

In a moment he attacked the left eye in the same manner. When he was done, he patted the boy and told him to get off the table. The boy got down, blinked his eyes, stared around him, then lifted his hands and looked at them, one after the other. His mother rushed to him and they both began to cry as he saw her face for the first time.

Brazil has other healers, all equally adept at miracles. Palmério is a healer who does not attempt surgery, but cures by the laying on of hands. Isaltina is a mystic who also cures by touch, influencing the "fluid" of the patients. By a curious coincidence she too is possessed by the spirit of a German doctor, indicating, perhaps, the respect with which Brazilians view the many German emigrants to their country. This doctor is named Artz Scovsk: he appeared to her in a trance and told her he had "unfinished business" for which he intended to use her as a medium.

Isaltina's most famous case was the restoration to health of the former secretary to the governor of Rio Grande do Norte, himself a doctor, but badly crippled. This procedure, it is said, was broadcast live on television and monitored by seven physicians from the best hospitals in Rio de Janeiro.

Chapter 6

FAITH HEALERS

And when the day of Pentecost was fully come,
They were all with one accord in one place.
And suddenly there was a sound from Heaven
As of a rushing mighty wind, and it filled
All the house where they were sitting.
And there appeared unto them
Cloven tongues like as of fire,
And it sat upon each of them,
And they were all filled with the Holy Ghost,
And began to speak with other tongues,
As the Spirit gave them utterance.

ACTS II: 1-4,
KING JAMES VERSION

Faith healers are not lacking in our own country. Currently there has been a surge in the Pentecostal movement that appears to be spreading through the major Christian churches. It is estimated that in the U.S. some 300,000 Catholics have turned charismatic, and at least 100,000 Protestants.

Pentecostals believe in baptism during prayer meetings, to receive the power of the Holy Ghost. The sign that baptism has effectively taken place is the ability to "speak in tongues," or glossolalia, which describes an ecstatic utterance, usually unintelligible to the hearers or even the speaker himself.

Speaking in tongues is one of the nine gifts of the Spirit mentioned by St. Paul. The other eight are the interpretation of tongues, prophecy, the discerning of spirits, wisdom, knowledge, faith, healing, and miracles.

The laying on of hands is practiced en masse by Pentecostals, or by more professional practitioners like Oral Roberts or R. W. Schambach. Fundamentalist preachers and evangelists like Kathryn Kuhlman are liberally credited with healing miracles. Miss Kuhlman began preaching at the age of sixteen after the usual spiritual revelation, interpreted as a call, and a few years later was ordained by the Evangelical Church Alliance.

Her sessions draw scores of people who claim they have been healed of cancer, heart ailments, arthritis, deafness, and many kinds of pain. At a typical service she will touch the faces of those who come up to her, after which they often collapse into the arms of her aides, "under the power of the Holy Spirit." At any session there are likely to be people who arise from wheelchairs and walk, and those who throw away their crutches. The skeptics point out that there is no medical verification of these cures, or even of the original condition. For example, one woman who said she had been cured of heart disease, told a *New York Times* reporter after the service [1] that she, not her physician, had made the diagnosis of heart disease.

Miss Kuhlman works out of headquarters in a Pittsburgh hotel suite, where she tapes a daily half-hour radio program heard on fifty stations. She also tapes a television program in Los Angeles, which is seen on more than sixty TV stations. Her appearances bring in almost $2 million a year. She accepts a yearly salary of $25,000, plus travel expenses, turning the rest over to a nonprofit charitable foundation named after her.

She acknowledges that often enough her cures have failed, and there is much she does not understand. "I just don't know," she says.

Better known than Kathryn Kuhlman is evangelist Oral Roberts, who has built an empire in Tulsa, Oklahoma, which includes a university, a home for the aged, a publishing company, an ongoing television program, a computer center, and a direct mail operation.

Oral Roberts dislikes the term "faith healer." "It suggests that

[1] *New York Times,* October 20, 1972.

I'm doing the healing rather than God." His intercession, how-ever, is apparently necessary. He claims to have laid hands on more than a million suffering heads. With all that, he has had his share of failure.

"I know how many I've prayed for who, when I finished pray-ing, looked up in hurt and disappointment because nothing had happened. My failures are ever before me." [2]

On the other hand, he is credited with having healed large numbers of people. The question which remains open, as always, is what constitutes a cure, and how permanent is it?

Early in his career, Roberts earned little respect outside Pen-tecostal circles. Today his operations make those of Kathryn Kuhlman look like small time. His annual budget is $17 million. He has a weekly half-hour television program that goes to 275 stations in the U.S. and Canada. Four times a year he puts on a TV special that costs $600,000, and is carried by more than 400 stations. He publishes a magazine called *Abundant Life*. The Oral Roberts University in Tulsa has an ultra-modern campus valued at $55 million, offers full academic accreditation, and has a good basketball team.

He operates a home for the aged, and a mail order service called the Oral Roberts Association which employs 300 people and carries a mailing load of 400,000 letters a month, a large share of which consists of advice on personal problems and answers to requests for prayer.

Like virtually every other evangelist, Roberts heard a direct call from God to assume his preaching. At the age of seventeen he had collapsed during a basketball game with blood running from his nose and was carried home, apparently near death from an advanced case of tuberculosis. He languished for six months and then his sister took him to George Moncey, an obscure tent evangelist, who laid hands on him and asked Christ to open his lungs.

The miracle happened. A sensation of warmth came over him and penetrated his lungs. He took the first deep breath he'd had in months, and talked without stammering, an affliction he'd had since childhood. Then he heard the voice: "You are to take my healing power to your generation."

[2] *New York Times Magazine*, April 22, 1973.

Roberts was ordained in the Pentecostal Holiness Church, a small, independent sect, which emphasizes mystical experiences, such as speaking in tongues. He preached in Enid, Oklahoma, for a while, but became dissatisfied that he was not reaching the whole man in praying only for the soul, and began praying to heal the body as well.

In 1968 he left the Pentecostal movement and joined the Methodist Church. Headquarters is now the Oral Roberts University. He receives $24,000 a year in salary and puts his book royalties into a trust fund for his children. He is rated as a shrewd businessman in Tulsa, with an impressive record in assessing real-estate potential. He is said to be interested in obtaining a charter for an Oral Roberts bank in Tulsa.

Roberts's critics make the charges which can be levied at all evangelists: oversimplification of problems, concentration on one-self rather than social responsibilities, and interpreting religion as a kind of supermarket where you can buy progress through positive thinking, do-it-yourself psychology, send-us-a-contribu-tion-and-God-will-reward-you-with-prosperity kind of appeal.

His failures in healing trouble him, but on very different grounds than would affect a medical man. To Roberts it is tied in with the strength of faith, to the physician with his own short-comings in knowledge.

Of all the faith-healing movements, one of the most influential is Christian Science, founded by Mary Baker Eddy in 1866. The basic premise on which Mrs. Eddy founded the Christian Science Church, and her attitude toward illness, was that the "mortal mind produces all disease."

Obviously, what the mind creates, the mind can abolish. The founder herself sometimes hedged her bets. When questioned about some dental work she was having done with anesthesia, she replied that refusal to cooperate fully with the dentist would turn his mental protest against her, so that "his mental force weighs against a painless operation, whereas it should be put into the same scale as mine, thus producing a painless operation as a logical result." [3]

Similarly, when challenged for wearing spectacles, she replied that she "wore glasses because of the sins of the world." If you

[3] *Christian Science Today*, Charles S. Braden, Southern Methodist University Press, Dallas, Texas, 1958.

weigh the ambiguity of the first answer against the heads-I-win-tails-you-lose quality of the second answer, you may find it difficult to conceive of her losing an argument.

The philosophy of the Christian Science movement appears to be contained in Mrs. Eddy's "Scientific Statement of Being." This statement declares: "There is no life, truth, intelligence nor substance in matter. All is infinite Mind and its infinite manifestation, for God is All-in-all. Spirit is immortal Truth; matter is mortal error. Spirit is the real and eternal; matter is the unreal and temporal. Spirit is God, and man is His image and likeness. Therefore man is not material; he is spiritual." [4]

If God is good, evil could not be created by God, and therefore must be unreal. Sin, sickness, and death appear in human experience only because unrealities are made to seem real by errors in belief. (It is very difficult to suppress the notion at this point that without a single exception people eventually make the error of dying, Mrs. Eddy among them, but perhaps this is an unworthy thought.) The fact is that illness, represented by mental and bodily disharmony, is illusion. Man, reflecting the spirit of his Maker, is incapable of sin, sickness, and death.

If matter possesses nothing of life, truth, intelligence, nor substance, Mrs. Eddy asks, can it feel or think? The answer is no, the brain does not think, the nerves do not feel. There is no matter, and there is no mortal mind either, although in other places and at other times she speaks of mortal mind that understands. Mind understands, and this precludes the need of believing; the body, being matter, cannot believe, but the belief and the believer are one, being mortal.

All clear?

The way to cure a patient is to show him that his disease is unreal. Mortal mind produces disease through fear. Remove the fear and end the disease.

Man as a harmonious being is incapable of suffering, of feeling pain, of being sick, or even of being thirsty. Symptoms of disease are only evidence of false belief, hence the road to cure is by arguing that man is innately perfect. And, since the material body is only a mental concept, the disease is destroyed by showing the patient that it is impossible for matter to suffer or to feel

[4] *Science and Health,* Christian Science Publications, Boston, Mass., 1906.

pain. According to Mrs. Eddy, "a sick body is evolved from sick thoughts." [5] The patient needs to be instructed out of this "illusion of sickness."

One might assume from this that it is the patient's awakened faith that will cure him, yet in another work [6] Mrs. Eddy promotes the idea that the patient need not be convinced at all—"if the healer realizes the truth, it will free his patient."

In Braden's book he relates asking a practitioner about this point and, assuming he had an infected finger, asking what the practitioner would do? The answer was, "I would *know* that your finger was perfect. Seeing it as God sees it and so knowing it, it would be well."

"But," Braden asked, "suppose I go on thinking it is there, even when you know it isn't? What then?"

"It doesn't make any difference what you think. When I know it is not there, it is healed. It is the knowing of the practitioner that determines the healing. It does not depend upon the belief or the faith of the patient."

One might leap to the conclusion that this would make failure impossible, since the practitioners must be presumed secure in their belief, even if the patient is not. But since there are failures, it is evident that even practitioners are all too human.

Today's practicing physician does not underestimate the power of faith, suggestion, psychology, tender loving care, or whatever you wish to call it. He knows how large a share it plays in any cure. In the treatment of pain it plays, perhaps, a major part. But as medical historian Dr. Howard W. Haggard says, "The procedure of . . . the medicine man relieves pain, but it heals no broken legs, nor does it cure measles or smallpox or cancer. It takes the pain from an aching tooth, but it fills no cavity." [7]

[5] *Science and Health.*
[6] *Rudimental Divine Science*, E. J. F. Eddy, Boston, Mass., 1893.
[7] *The Lame, the Halt and the Blind*, Harper & Brothers, New York, 1932.

Chapter 7

THE PAIN CLINIC

To run a pain clinic you have to be obsessive and you have to be persistent.

DR. JOHN J. BONICA

During World War II, Dr. John J. Bonica was stationed at a large army hospital in the West as chief of anesthesiology.

"Early in 1944," he recalled, "we were getting waves and waves of people coming from the Pacific with a variety of injuries, particularly nerve injuries which produced causalgia and other reflex dystrophies."

Reflex sympathetic dystrophies are disorders of the sympathetic nervous system which may follow injury. In addition to severe pain, they can lead to serious disability, with weakness and changes in muscles, bones, joints, and skin. The hospital was an orthopedic center and received many wounded soldiers in great pain from orthopedic conditions resulting from their injuries. The first problem was to stop the pain.

"I had heard during my training in New York," Dr. Bonica said, "that Dr. E. A. Rovenstine was using nerve blocks, which is a method whereby a local anesthetic is injected around a nerve to produce anesthesia. He used these blocks to relieve chronic pain states. I became interested in this and looked at the litera-

ture, and of course realized that it went back to about 1879, even
before Karl Koller demonstrated the anesthetic activity of cocaine for surgical anesthesia. Cocaine was then used for the relief
of chronic pain of tuberculosis of the larynx and various other
conditions."

Nerve block, as Dr. Bonica later detailed in his book, *The Management of Pain,* goes back a great deal farther. In fact, if you
consider acupuncture a form of nerve block, the Chinese were
using it as early as 3000 B.C. In the Western world there were
attempts at injecting an opiate to relieve pain as early as 1665.
The French surgeon LaFargue was quite successful in 1836 in
injecting morphine paste subcutaneously and relieving pain.

The invention of the syringe and needle in 1852 by C. Pravaz
in Paris was an important breakthrough, although credit for this
invention is usually given to A. Wood of Edinburgh, who seems
to have invented it independently in 1855 and did a better job of
publicizing it.

In any case, it was Karl Koller who, in 1884, used cocaine to
demonstrate the value of regional analgesia. Cocaine interrupted
the messages traveling along the nerves without injuring the
nerve itself. In some cases this was desirable, where only a temporary effect was needed. But where the pain consistently returned as the drug wore off, it was a disadvantage.

In 1900, a German surgeon named H. Schlösser experimented
with alcohol injected into the fifth cranial nerve to relieve the
intense pain of trigeminal neuralgia, a facial neuralgia.

Alcohol destroyed the nerve and brought much more lasting
relief. Even where there was regeneration of the nerve tissue,
where all the cells had not been destroyed, and the nerve grew
back, follow-up shots again brought long-lasting relief.

Dr. Bonica began to use the technique of nerve block and was
successful in some situations, but found many cases were not that
easily solved, and that puzzling problems remained.

He took his problems to a neurosurgeon at the hospital, then
talked to an orthopedic surgeon, and eventually widened the
discussion to include a psychiatrist.

"Now I realized that trying to work in the usual traditional
way in which I might refer a case to the orthopedic surgeon and
he would see the patient in his clinic, and then he would write a

note on the chart, and then I would try to interpret his note—
that bothered me. Often, after reading his note, I would go to
his office and say, 'I'd like to talk to you more about this.'

"And soon it came about that I was getting these people together in conferences, informal conferences, and found that this
interaction and personal exchange was effective when it cleared
many things up for us. So I began to talk about this pain clinic
concept.

"About this time, independently and unknowingly, a Dr. Dun-
can Alexander, who had worked with Dr. Rovenstine in New
York, was doing the same thing in the army and subsequently
in a Veterans' Administration Hospital in Texas."

After the war, Dr. Bonica and Dr. Alexander got together and
had long conversations in which they discussed the tantalizing
problems and their own sense of inadequacy. They quickly
agreed that the attack on pain had to become a team effort.

Dr. Bonica began writing articles, which were published in
American journals and widely abroad in France, Italy, Germany,
Scandinavia, Britain, Canada, and South America.

He realized too that there was no comprehensive source of
information dealing with all aspects of pain, and how valuable
such a compilation would be. A plan for a book began to evolve.

Upon leaving the army he went into private practice in Tacoma, Washington. He had kept records of the many patients he
had treated and he continued to exert both interest and effort
in the treatment of pain; this attracted chronic pain patients
from all over the country. "I tried to continue this pain clinic
conference concept. There was a fine neurosurgeon I worked
with, one or two psychiatrists (although they weren't too much
interested), and a few internists. But in private practice there
are many obstacles which I think hamper this kind of team effort. People are busy, they have their office hours, and there are
many other problems.

"Anyway, when I came to the University of Washington in
1960, I found Dr. Lowell White, a neurosurgeon, was also interested in pain, so I discussed the concept with him. And in the
meantime I had written the book."

Dr. Bonica's book, *The Management of Pain*, published in
1953, is a monumental work of 1,533 pages. It took him four years

to write, four years of intense, single-minded effort, blocking out all other activities except his practice.

"It was an incredible, obsessive kind of schedule. Eight P.M. to three o'clock in the morning, every single day. Saturday, eight A.M. to midnight. Sunday, eight A.M. to midnight. This went on for four years."

On top of that, he continued his practice. "From seven in the morning to six at night, I was down there at Tacoma General, leading a very active anesthesia program."

But despite the writing and the talking—"I almost pleaded with people that this was a good idea"—it was largely ignored until about 1970. And then, like other ideas whose time has come, there was a great surge of interest, and pain clinics began to sprout in many parts of the world.

Writing of pain clinics in England, Dr. Mark Swerdlow* whose own work in this field goes back to 1949, notes there are now such clinics in many of the big cities in Great Britain and credits Dr. Bonica's contributions in the field.[1]

Another English investigator, M. D. Churcher,** discussing nerve blocks,[2] likewise refers to the Bonica book, which has become the standard reference since its publication.

Of the many pain clinics now operating, the one at University Hospital in Seattle under Dr. Bonica's direction is the prototype. With Dr. Richard G. Black as coordinator it is possibly the best organized and most experienced, as well as the best known.

There is an important pain center at the City of Hope National Medical Center in Duarte, California. Dr. Crue, Chairman of the Division of Clinical Neurology and Director of the Department of Neurosurgery, is a man intensely interested in the neurophysiology of pain. He holds a number of important staff appointments at other hospitals in the southern California area, as well as teaching appointments. Over the past several years he has produced, with various collaborators, many scientific papers on

* M.D., M.Sc., FFARCS, Department of Anesthesia, Salford Hospitals Group, Manchester, England.
[1] "The Pain Clinic," *British Journal of Clinical Practice*, Vol. 26, No. 9, September 1972, pp. 403-7.
** M.B., B.S., FFARCS, Anesthetist, Plymouth General Hospital, Plymouth, England.
[2] "Pain Clinics," *The Practitioner*, Vol. 204, February 1970, pp. 273-5.

pain and has edited a book titled *Pain and Suffering: Selected Aspects.*[3]

Dr. Richard Sternbach, whose specialty is the psychology of pain, is doing pioneering work at the Veterans' Administration Hospital in San Diego and the University of California San Diego School of Medicine in La Jolla.

Dr. Ronald L. Katz, formerly Professor of Anesthesiology at Columbia University's College of Physicians and Surgeons in New York, had begun organizing a formal pain clinic at Columbia, but in the summer of 1973 moved to Los Angeles to become Chairman of the Department of Anesthesiology at UCLA Medical Center, where he is setting up a full-scale pain clinic. In New York, Dr. Lester Mark and Dr. Herbert Spiegel, who worked with Dr. Katz, are continuing the work of organizing a pain clinic for Columbia.

The headache unit at Montefiore Hospital in New York has become nationally known through the work of its Physician-in-Charge, Dr. Arnold Friedman, who is also Clinical Professor of Neurology at Columbia. Dr. Friedman, who writes and lectures extensively, intends to devote himself full-time to teaching.

The Pain Rehabilitation Center at La Crosse, Wisconsin, under the direction of Dr. C. Norman Shealy, has done important work in electrical stimulation for the control of pain, and there are many others: Dr. Henry K. Beecher of Harvard Medical School, Dr. Edward R. Perl of the University of North Carolina Medical School, Dr. Arthur Taub of the Yale School of Medicine, and dozens of others. There are pain clinics now in Japan, Great Britain, Germany, Brazil, Uruguay, and Venezuela.

An international symposium on pain held in Seattle in May 1973, sponsored by the University of Washington School of Medicine and the National Institutes of Health, and supported by funds from both government and industry, drew 102 participants from all over the world, with 86 speakers presenting scientific papers on new research in pain control. In addition to the American doctors present, participants came from Canada, Sweden, England, France, Scotland, Germany, Russia, Japan, Italy, Holland, and Czechoslovakia.

After years of Dr. Bonica's exhorting and preaching, the idea

[3] Charles C. Thomas, Springfield, Ill., 1970.

is taking hold that the treatment of chronic pain is a complex affair that requires the combined attention of a team of specialists —a true multidisciplinary effort. "As specialization in the medical profession becomes greater and greater," he says, "and we develop what I like to refer to as narrower and narrower tubular vision, it is absolutely essential to have these kinds of team effort in taking care of patients, in teaching, and in research."

What is team effort at a pain clinic? As Dr. Richard Black, the Seattle pain clinic coordinator, explains it, "Unless there is a team approach, the patient can be bounced from internist to orthopedist to neurologist to psychiatrist and back again, endlessly. This happens unless their work is coordinated, unless there is a team approach. They've got to talk to each other."

The pain clinic at the University of Washington hospital came into being when Dr. Bonica joined forces with Dr. White. They began to see chronic pain patients and to hold fairly regular meetings. Slowly they enlisted help from others—orthopedists, internists, surgeons, pharmacologists, psychiatrists, psychologists, and other specialists.

As the pain clinic became more formalized, rules were born of necessity. Every doctor who joined the group had to have a special interest in chronic pain; he had to have particular knowledge of pain syndromes; he had to be skilled in diagnosis and have a contribution to make to therapy; and he had to be willing to devote the considerable time and effort—often at a personal sacrifice—that the job required.

Today the pain clinic at Seattle is made up of twenty-two specialists in many different disciplines. These include: anesthesiology, general surgery, internal medicine, neurology, neurosurgery, oral surgery, orthopedics, physical medicine, pharmacology, psychiatry, psychology, radiology, and neurophysiology. In addition to the specialists there are two nurses, a sociologist, and a social worker.

Patients accepted at the pain clinic must be referred by a physician. The number that can be accepted is limited, and there is a backlog waiting to be admitted. Every patient is thoroughly screened to make sure that he actually requires the multidiscipline approach, or whether he can be treated in one of the regular hospital clinics with an expenditure of considerably less time, money, and energy. The patients accepted at the pain clinics are those with tough problems that have not yielded to ordinary clinical therapy.

Screening begins with a physician after all the medical records of the patient have been collected and reviewed by the pain clinic staff. With the medical history reviewed and assessed, and preliminary agreement reached that this patient seems to need the pain clinic approach, the next step is an interview with a staff physician. Everything available: X-rays, tests, previous consultations, operations if any—all have been studied and evaluated. This is not only part of the screening, it avoids duplicating costly or unpleasant tests or other procedures that might otherwise be prescribed.

The patient may have been asked to keep a two-week record on a form supplied by the clinic, which charts his time in or out of bed, and his general level of activity. At the time of admission he is asked to write a two-page description of the pain, his family history, and other personal details.

The patient is assigned a physician for the interview who will also become his personal manager at the clinic. This doctor performs the initial examination and work-up, makes decisions about which consultants to see, and acts as liaison between the patient, the doctors of the pain clinic, and the patient's own personal physician.

From the examination, the patient's medical history, and the initial interview with his physician-manager, a detailed description of the pain problem is made up. A psychiatric profile, the MMPI, or Minnesota Multiple Personality Inventory, is also obtained. The MMPI offers a guide to the patient's score in such behavior tendencies as the hysterical, the hypochondriacal, obsessive-compulsive, depressive, masculine-feminine, schizophrenic, and other categories, all or any of which affect his responses to the pain experience. His scoring in answer to selected questions helps flag a warning as to possible abnormal reactions.

The first question the examining physician must decide is whether or not there is any physical basis for the pain. A patient who has scored high in hypochondria or hysteria may have pain that has no physical basis at all. This does not mean the pain is not real. It is real, and it can hurt just as much as a crushed finger, but the treatment must necessarily be different.

So part of the initial assessment is a complete physical examination. The physician can then determine what kinds of tests, X-rays, and consultations appear to be needed. A decision is also made at this time whether to hospitalize the patient or permit him to come in for treatment as an outpatient, continuing to live at home.

There is, of course, an advantage to a week's hospitalization, during which all the tests can be run off. But this is balanced by the advantage of the outpatient method in seeing the patient at intervals over a period of weeks. The problem with chronic pain is that it may vary widely in intensity over any given period of time. Patients are warned that their pain may subside as soon as they are admitted to the clinic, or it may become more severe. The staff is interested in any fluctuation and in seeing the patient at the times pain is bad, and at the times it is mild.

The pain clinic's function is purely diagnostic. Once some kind of decision as to treatment is reached, the patient is referred to the appropriate center for actual therapy, either in the hospital, or back to his personal physician.

The diagnosis, once established, and the mechanism of the pain determined, recommendations for treatment must be laid out very carefully. At least five factors must be considered, according to Dr. Bonica:

1. The cause of the pain, its location, path, and mechanism, its intensity and probable duration.
2. The nature of the disease (if any) causing the pain.
3. Age of the patient, physical and mental condition, life expectancy, obligations to family and community.
4. Treatment methods available locally, and practical under the prevailing circumstances.
5. Complications and side effects that might develop as a result of treatment.

Half measures are to be shunned; unless the physician is prepared to spend a great deal of time and effort, he cannot hope to do any good—he may do more harm than good. The most common reason for failure is insufficient time spent on the patient. Many patients require the concentrated efforts of their physician and one or more specialists who are brought in to contribute their particular skill and knowledge.

The keystone of this approach in the pain clinic is the weekly conference. This is when patients with particular problems, for whom diagnosis or therapy has not been decided, are presented to all the members of the group for a round-robin discussion.

During the normal hour and a half of each conference, two patients are usually considered. A synopsis of each case is distributed beforehand to all the members of the group. The director, Dr. Bonica, or the clinic coordinator, Dr. Black, is chairman of the session. The patient's manager presents a summary of the medical history and physical findings, and asks the consultants who have been brought into the case to add their comments and opinions. The other specialists can then ask questions and make comments.

At some point the patient, and usually his spouse, is brought in to answer further questions and to ask questions of their own of the group. When the patient leaves, the medical discussion goes on until some sort of decision as to diagnosis and therapy is reached, or it is determined that no decision can be made from the data so far available.

The following two case studies are fairly typical:

CASE HISTORY ONE

Mr. S is a white male, forty-two years old, with a five-year history of low-back pain. The pain began when he strained his back in June 1968 lifting a heavy object; pain developed in the lumbosacral region on the left side. Some weeks of rest helped, and he seemed to have recovered, although he still had some residual pain.

Several months later he developed urinary tract symptoms which led to an operation. He thought the surgery also helped his back pain.

In 1969 the back pain returned with severe pain in the left leg. A myelogram, or X-ray of the spine, showed a herniated disk and in June 1969 an operation was performed to remove an extruded fragment.

Three days after the operation he experienced increasing pain with numbness in the left leg. Another operation was performed to decompress the vertebra, and this appeared to relieve the leg pain.

He returned to work, but within three months was forced to quit by a recurrence of back pain. In October 1969, he was placed in a cast for a month and taken off medication. He seemed to gain relief. He then went to another physician who performed another myelogram and then carried out another operation for some type of fusion of the lower back.

The second operation did not help the pain, which had become steady and severe. He was admitted to the orthopedic service of the hospital in June 1972 and referred to the pain clinic.

He described the pain as feeling like a spear coming from above the site of the incision in his back and radiating into both legs and the left foot. The pain was so intense that it produced nausea and gagging, and gave him headaches.

Physical examination of Mr. S showed him well developed and well nourished, but agitated and confused. There was marked muscle spasm in the back, with decreased movement of the lower spine. There was tenderness in several areas, but no significant motor loss, and all reflexes were functioning.

He had had consultations in orthopedics, anesthesiology, physical medicine, and psychiatry. He had had three trials with the transcutaneous stimulator. This is an electrical apparatus which sends a low current through the skin and, for reasons not yet understood (unless it be a loading of the large fibers à la Melzack-Wall gate hypothesis), appears to bring temporary relief of pain to a significant number of chronic pain patients. In Mr. S's case, the electrodes were tried on his lower back and also on his right hand. The result was relief of pain for several hours, the effect much more marked when the electrodes were placed on the back than on the hand.

The discussion began before Mr. S was brought into the conference room. Dr. Fordyce, psychologist, mentioned that the patient was extremely contrary. He insisted he had a photographic memory and, in his last interview, deliberately answered questions completely opposite to the answers he had given in a previous interview.

Offered various programs of therapy, he played the "Yes, but—" game, finding an objection to every suggestion made. He flatly turned down any invitation to come into the hospital's rehabilitation center.

He told a story of beating up his son, whom he had caught with marijuana in his possession; when the police refused to arrest the boy, he took him to the police station and dumped him in front of the building.

Dr. Herbert Ripley, psychiatrist-in-chief, had also seen Mr. S. He had heard the story about the son and the marijuana with additional details. Mr. S said he had also beaten up a couple of his son's friends and frightened them by firing his pistol near them. He boasted about being a crack shot, talked continually about violence and fighting. His wife, when interviewed, had said she thought he was suicidal—he had talked about it, and that she was afraid of him.

Dr. Ripley gave his opinion that Mr. S needed psychiatric treatment, that he was unpredictable, and that there was depression underlying the hostility. He had responded to two drugs: Mellaril, a tranquilizer, and Elavil, an antidepressant, seeming calmer after taking them.

Dr. Black, clinic coordinator, thought the scope of the reports offered insufficient grounds on which to base a course of treatment. The experiment with the transcutaneous stimulator had apparently provided relief of pain; was it a placebo effect?

But the interpretation of the group was mixed. Did Mr. S get enough relief to warrant being given one of the stimulators to take home? If it relieved his pain, could he be considered cured?

There was a short discussion about the advisability of giving him a "black box" to take home, with general agreement that this would not be enough. There were other problems.

Dr. Fordyce felt that Mr. S was working too hard at holding on to his illness. Dr. Ripley agreed and made it more forceful. The man was psychotic, Dr. Ripley felt. He clung to his illusions, his machismo. He rode a motorcycle when he could, and went out on gopher shooting trips. Even though he had suddenly "gotten religion," Dr. Ripley felt he might be dangerous, citing his wife's fear of him.

The question remained, what to do? They couldn't keep him indefinitely at the pain clinic. Perhaps he should be sent back to the hospital from which he was referred. He seemed to like the resident psychiatrist there, perhaps that doctor could help him.

At this point Mr. S was brought in. He was wearing a hospital robe and sitting on a wheeled stretcher. He appeared calm but watchful, his eyes moving from doctor to doctor. He answered their questions willingly and respectfully.

Asked about the transcutaneous stimulator, he said it helped—felt like pinpricks on the skin, not pleasant, but it did relieve the pain for a while. He didn't sleep well, got up and walked around a lot. Standing was better than lying down. He described the pain as a deep, tearing sensation. He told a story about a dog that had annoyed him—he would have shot her, always carried a gun, but denied that he would ever shoot anyone, presumably a human.

Mr. S was taken out. Dr. Fordyce picked up his chart and said there had been no essential change. Mr. S was a very disturbed, confused man. Recommended treatment would require more study, more data than they had so far.

CASE HISTORY TWO

Mr. B was an airplane pilot, a crop duster, thirty-six years old. He had had two airplane accidents. The first, in 1967, resulted in fractures of the spine. He wore a brace, but two years later complained of low-back pain, with radiation to the leg. Myelogram showed defects in the vertebrae and, in May 1969, he had an operation for the removal of several disks.

He returned to work and, in September 1969, had a second plane crash. His back pains increased, and the pain continued to radiate down the left leg. He had a second operation to remove portions of damaged vertebrae, with spinal fusion.

Pain and radiation to the legs continued, with a sensation of numbness and a feeling of cold in the legs. He also experienced bowel and bladder urgency, but no incontinence.

Physical examination showed restricted trunk movement, a limitation on leg raising, knee-jerk reflexes normal, but ankle jerks reduced. There was no motor weakness, but the sensory level showed a loss.

Mr. B had had consultations in orthopedics, neurosurgery, and psychiatry. His medication had included Talwin for pain and Valium for relief of tension and anxiety. These were discontinued and he was then getting only Percodan for pain.

Mr. B was not available for the conference, and the discussion went on without him. Dr. Fordyce offered the opinion that his psychological profile, as indicated by the MMPI, suggested emotional factors, despite the very real injuries in Mr. B's case. He came through as bitter, frustrated, tense, and somatic (the latter is a psychiatric term that means that emotional conflicts are converted into physical symptoms). Dr. Fordyce had doubts that a change in environment would have a significant effect on Mr. B's pain.

Dr. Stewart, orthopedic surgeon, felt that Mr. B's symptoms did not fully tie in with his history. He had good reason for pain, but what was his reaction to it? Was it over and beyond what one might reasonably expect? Admittedly, some people with spinal fractures do develop delayed symptoms. And the myelograms did show a widening of space between some segments of the vertebrae, which can produce increased pressure by encroaching on the canal. Yet no encroachment was visible, and no pathology. The widening did not seem to account for the pain, and surgery would not be an answer. Mr. B, he thought, had more than enough fusion of his back; any more would leave him no mobility at all in his spine.

Dr. Ripley thought Mr. B was not psychotic. Some depression was to be expected with so much pain. He seemed a stable enough personality. The group agreed that conservative management was to be recommended, including a program of planned exercise and psychological encouragement.

The meeting disbanded, and Dr. Stewart offered some general thoughts. "Low-back pain," he said, "is almost a social disease. It's like a clue to something much broader. These patients tend to have more mental problems, more alcoholism, and similar troubles.

"And yet, low-back pain is so common with us that it may be a natural result of our upright postures, part of the way we live. In India, the only ruptured disk problems are among the visiting foreigners. Indians don't stand around to talk, they squat on their heels, which is easier on the spine. From an anatomical standpoint, much sitting is also bad. It compresses the disks in the spine."

In another chapter we shall have a further look at low-back pain as a chronic pain problem, and a social disease, and see what new understanding has been gained and what new approaches are being used in its treatment.

Chapter 8

DRUGS AGAINST PAIN

The opiates do not kill pain. They change people's interpretation of pain—treat their suffering, not their pain.

Dr. Lawrence M. Halpern [*]

The usual reaction to pain is to look for something to swallow to make it go away. Frequently enough if you swallow the right pill and the pain is uncomplicated and transient, it works well enough. It is also simple, easy, and cheap. But there is room for error—the wrong drug, the wrong dosage, or too much of a good thing—overuse.

Pain does not always require an analgesic. The pain may be coming from an infection, in which case an antibiotic could be the correct treatment, or from arthritis, in which case an anti-inflammatory agent would provide better relief than an analgesic, although it happens that aspirin is both. Pain stemming from anxiety and tension may call for a sedative or a muscle relaxant, rather than a pain killer as such.

There are many drugs that are useful for pain on a short-term basis. With long and sustained use, problems may arise. The ideal analgesic has yet to be discovered, the drug that acts powerfully against pain but has no side effects and is not addictive. Hope

[*] Associate Professor, Department of Pharmacology; member, Pain Clinic, University of Washington School of Medicine, Seattle, Washington.

of discovering such a drug is what keeps the lights burning at night in pharmaceutical laboratories.

Still, analgesic and other drugs, properly used, are indispensable in the control of pain. As the pharmacologist of Seattle's pain clinic, Dr. Halpern takes a very down-to-earth approach to his specialty.

"When you have an acute pain situation—somebody breaks a leg, or somebody goes into the hospital for surgery—the problem of preoperative and postoperative management of pain is really a very simple thing.

"You premedicate the patient with some slow or fast dope and some sedative, take him up to the operating room and gas him until he's blind. When he doesn't see any more, you cut and fix and pull, and then you take him down and keep him stoned for two or three days, and at the end of two or three days you unstone him very quickly and he doesn't hurt any more. He gets up then and he's shocked by the size of the bill, and he goes home.

"And that's like 95 percent or 99 percent of the management of pain as it exists in the country. But the other couple of percent—I think that the figures Dr. Bonica gives for the chronic pain patient and the loss of time and effort in work is staggering. And while that's a very small percentage of patients actually, they are probably some of the most difficult people in the world to manage.

"So the short-term case is no problem. Any of several good analgesics will do the job. But the chronic pain patient is something else. Can you feed him drugs month after month, year after year?

"One of the things we've learned is that after about six weeks on opiates, on good strong analgesic drugs, you don't buy anything by continuing to medicate the patient. In fact, you're probably buying more problems than you started with. Problems in terms of side effects, in terms of the emotional changes in the patient, in terms of the fact that you do not cover the patient's pain with opiate/analgesic drugs after about six weeks.

"It's not so much the common idea that the pain becomes resistant to the drug. But the drug produces a variety of different kinds of effects than what we think of as analgesia. For instance, when you talk about morphine to people, they really don't have any concept of what morphine does, except that it blocks pain.

And the closest experience that most people have to blockaded pain is that they go to the dentist, he shoots some gunk down around the fifth nerve and blocks it and they're anesthetized, and that to them is what analgesia is—they don't feel pain.

"Morphine doesn't do that at all, because under the influence of an opiate/analgesic drug, people feel their pain. They just interpret it in a different way. It doesn't bother them, it doesn't worry them. They can go to sleep in pain. They're comfortable about pain.

"I came to understand this, first of all by reading about other people's descriptions of the opiate effect. And secondly, by burning myself very badly about four years ago and going into the operating room a couple of times to have my hand rebuilt, and experiencing severe pain and severe concern about other things having to do with the opiate.

"It's been known for years, for instance, that a man who has a heart attack will clutch his chest and fall to the ground in pain and then worry about the fact that he's dying, and kill himself in compensating. What you do if you happen to be walking by is that you give him a small dose of morphine intravenously, which has no effect at all on the heart or the circulation; all it does is to block his worry. He tells you that he still feels the pain in his chest—it's a little bit less accurate in terms of definition than before, but it doesn't bother him any more, and that's what saves his life. The opiates change people's interpretation of pain. The opiates treat their suffering, not their pain.

"Up until a hundred years ago, morphine was called God's own medicine. It was the best, most efficient tranquilizer that anybody ever knew. Heroin—that's diacetylmorphine—is used for the same reason. It makes the junkies feel that much better. It makes their suffering go away, and for a little while they are able to cope.

"There are groups of people we think of as hypochondriacs who crave this kind of feeling of normality, of relief from the anxiety and the fears. That's the kind of action this drug has. And surprisingly enough, in none of the neurophysiological tests that have been done on this compound has anybody ever shown that it does block the reception or the transmission of pain in standard neuro-anatomical pathways. So whatever the opiates do, it's high and it's central (in the nervous system).

"The other side of the coin is that the opiates have a bunch of side effects that raise problems. *Addiction is not a problem per se.* The development of physical dependence is handled very, very easily, and it's just not a problem with the iatrogenic addict (condition or illness resulting from the treatment itself).

"We make people addicted who are dependent on drugs all the time. We detoxify them and very few, if any, wind up on the street shooting heroin.

"Heroin on the street is a behavior effect. We have a problem though, convincing many people who come from good, God-fearing, Bible-toting families. The opiate that they are taking for pain is indeed going to make them dependent upon it for relief during the time they are being treated. This is not a sign of weakness, nor should they equate it with addiction.

"There has been a tremendous overkill in terms of the concern about addiction. *Addiction is not a problem,* except an economic problem for the people who are deprived of their drug. Some of the side effects of the opiates are a problem, but the addiction per se is not a problem.

"It's not a problem as long as the patient can get his medicine. We give people methadone on the street, they're no longer a problem. If a physician keeps prescribing medicine for his patient, but the patient continues to have pain, the pain is going to be a problem, not the medicine.

"There is such hysteria about addiction in this country that one of the prime reasons for the failure of an analgesic drug is that the local doctor doesn't give enough to get a full therapeutic effect because he's afraid of addicting the patient. What he's doing is responding like a layman and becoming afraid of the problem of addiction, and therefore is depriving his patient of the benefits of full and adequate doses of opiates at the time he needs them."

Dr. Halpern's opinion in this respect coincides with that of Dr. Nathan Kline, Director of the Research Center at Rockland State Hospital, Orangeburg, New York. Dr. Kline has said,[1] speaking particularly of psychotherapeutic drugs, that far from being an overmedicated society, as some scare propaganda would have it, we are actually an undermedicated society in the

---

[1] "The Under-Medicated Patient." (Lecture. Place and date of delivery unavailable.)

sense that people are frequently afraid to take the full dose prescribed, skip doses, or break off treatment prematurely and so fail to get the full therapeutic results they should. This view has been further corroborated by a study done at the National Institute of Mental Health,[2] which concludes that "the present outcry about the misprescribing and claimed overuse of drugs is the consequence of a lack of appreciation of the complexities of psychotherapeutic drug prescribing in private practice and an overreaction to the specter of drug abuse."

"So that's one of the problems," says Dr. Halpern. "Another is that you develop tolerance and, despite the fact that the patient is on high doses of opiate and becomes physically dependent, many times the pain doesn't go away. Because the pain doesn't go away, the patient begins to respond peculiarly, with intensified depression, with behavioral changes both to the opiate and to the pain situation.

"Pretty soon you've got a vicious cycle where the patient loves to get stoned—they talk about pain, they get drugged instead, and you've got a patient who's really consuming drugs in an addiction mode, who isn't really talking about pain any more. That's one of the problems.

"Another problem is the side effects. The most serious side effect of high doses of opiate is the fact that you get respiratory depression and people don't breathe very well any more. They turn blue and they look kind of funny, and they even stop breathing if you give them high doses.

"And a fourth problem is constipation. We had a patient, a seventy-one-year-old lady dying of metastatic carcinoma, whose chief concern was constipation. She's a nurse, her daughter is a nurse, and her daughter was up here two or three times a day trying to clean her out so she could be comfortable.

"Dr. Black and I did a very miraculous thing for that lady. I put her on methadone, he took her down and blocked her (nerve block) and as soon as he blocked her, I cut her methadone back 25 percent. She ran to the john in frank diarrhea and everybody felt we did a good thing. She went home smiling.

"That's all we could do for her—we couldn't cure the cancer.

2 Mitchell Balter, Ph.D., and Jerome Levine, M.D., "Character and Extent of Psychotherapeutic Drug Usage in the United States," National Institute of Mental Health, Bethesda, Md.

But we were able to handle that particular aspect of her pain/ drug problem by removing some drugs."

In deciding which drug to use, Dr. Halpern believes the physician should first differentiate among pain conditions caused by injury or burns (traumatic), infections or inflammation (pathophysiologic), or those resulting from psychological disturbances or disorders.

Where a psychological factor is obvious, or at least where there is pain with insufficient physiological cause, it becomes necessary to consider the emotional problem as well as the pain. Emotional changes resulting from the drugs themselves must also be considered. For example, the patient may continue to complain about pain as a tactic to continue to receive the drug upon which he has become dependent, without realizing it himself. And, says Dr. Halpern, the narcotic may partially compensate him for the pain, while withdrawing it from him may uncover hidden psychoses or neurotic behavior of long duration.

He outlines a useful guide [3] which divides analgesics into three main categories: nonaddictive, moderately addictive, and strongly addictive. The choice is dictated by the kind of pain, its intensity, duration, and distribution.

NONADDICTIVE ANALGESICS

For mild pain such as ordinary headaches, neuralgia, joint and muscle pains, the non-narcotic or fever-reducing drugs, such as plain aspirin, are usually sufficient. In fact he says, "Special aspirin preparations or other proprietary mixtures are usually little better than aspirin and are often much more costly. Their use should be reserved for patients who are allergic to, or cannot tolerate, aspirin."

Aspirin is still the standard against which new drugs are measured for effectiveness in relieving mild or moderate pain. Its side effects are relatively few compared to its benefits; in addition to relieving pain it reduces fever and inflammation, which is why it is recommended for such differing conditions as colds and arthritis.

[3] "Analgesics and Other Drugs for the Relief of Pain," *Postgraduate Medicine*, Vol. 53, No. 6, May 1973, pp. 91-100.

One or two tablets (0.3 to 0.6 gram) every four hours have been shown to produce maximum results. More than 0.6 gram does not increase aspirin's ability to control pain, but may extend the duration of action. Larger doses will increase the side effects, which include gastric upset and often a painless bleeding of the stomach lining. High doses can also produce a condition known as salicylism, with ringing or buzzing in the ears, headache, sweating, increased heartbeat, and rapid, shallow breathing. Still higher doses can produce more severe effects, including respiratory failure, cardiovascular collapse, and death.

Special preparations or mixtures of aspirin and other products do not appear to offer substantial advantages. Buffered aspirin has not been shown to act faster or last longer. Because aspirin is acid, buffering it with aluminum hydroxide or magnesium carbonate may reduce irritation of the stomach wall, but so will a few ounces of milk.

Coated aspirin was developed to prevent bleeding by delaying absorption until the tablet is through the stomach and into the small intestine. This would seem to be opposed to the "fast action" claimed for buffered aspirin, but is primarily aimed at people with ulcers or other vulnerable conditions. The coating, however, introduces variables in absorption rate which makes the action rather unpredictable.

Sustained release, or timed-release, aspirin may contain two to four times as much aspirin per tablet with the claimed advantage that it dissolves slowly so that a single dose may carry through the entire day, keeping blood levels constant and avoiding the ups and downs of periodic dosing. In practice the superiority of this procedure has yet to be demonstrated.

There are aspirin combinations such as APC tablets, which contain aspirin, phenacetin, and caffeine, often claimed to have greater potency for pain relief than aspirin alone. Available data do not show that APC is superior to aspirin alone.

Compounds related to aspirin include salicylamide, sodium salicylate, phenacetin, and acetaminophen. Salicylamide has been promoted as a substitute for patients who are allergic to aspirin, or who wish to avoid the stomach irritation and induced bleeding possible with large doses of aspirin. Its advantages do not seem to be clear-cut. Dr. Halpern believes it to be no more effective than a placebo for pain, and sees little evidence for its use.

A word here for placebo. To a measurable degree it works. The power of suggestion is strong enough so that if a patient receives a pill made of milk sugar which he thinks is medication, he will obtain some relief, sometimes considerable relief. Many studies have been done in this area, and placebos work, up to a point, and for a limited time. It cannot be said that they work as well as the real medication, but on the other hand they cannot be written off as having zero effect.

Sodium salicylamide is more soluble than aspirin, hence should act more rapidly in theory, but appears to be less effective than aspirin.

Phenacetin, widely used in headache preparations, is about equal to aspirin in reducing pain, not as good in reducing fever or inflammation, so is less useful for arthritis. Moreover, large amounts of phenacetin, taken over a long period of time, have an adverse effect on the red blood cells, reducing their oxygen-carrying capacity, producing a condition known as methemoglobinemia.

Acetaminophen, as a substitute for phenacetin, reduces the risk of methemoglobinemia and has been recommended for long-term use where aspirin cannot be used. For the reduction of pain and fever, acetaminophen appears to equal aspirin, but not in anti-inflammatory effect; hence it is less useful for rheumatoid arthritis.

Where the pain is caused entirely by inflammation, as in arthritis, an anti-inflammatory drug is more important than an analgesic. Phenylbutazone is used for acute flare-ups in short-term therapy, generally a week for gout, bursitis, or tendonitis. The short-term restriction is because of phenylbutazone's toxicity, which carries risk of agranulocytosis, or loss of white blood cells. This drug and its close relatives, aminopyrine and oxyphenbutazone, are not recommended for long-term chronic pain therapy.

A new drug named Tegretol (carbamazepine) has been found for subduing the intense pain of tic douloureux, one of the unhappily common forms of trigeminal neuralgia. It works in about 75 percent of cases, but must be carefully monitored as it carries a risk of agranulocytosis and aplastic anemia. The manufacturer's warning emphasizes that Tegretol should not be considered a simple analgesic and should never be taken casually for the relief of trivial facial aches or pains.

Indocin (indomethacin) is a specialized anti-inflammatory agent specific for osteoarthritis of the hip, although it is also recommended for gout and ankylosing spondylitis, a kind of arthritis of the spine.

There has been controversy over Indocin, some critics maintaining it is no more effective than aspirin. Dr. Halpern says, "In terms of the analgesia produced in nonrheumatic pain, 50 mg. of indomethacin has been found to be approximately comparable to 600 mg. of aspirin." But long-term use of indomethacin, he says, is to be avoided because of adverse effects on the central nervous system and stomach. Used for the common forms of rheumatoid arthritis, results have been disappointing.

MODERATELY ADDICTIVE DRUGS

Best known in this group is codeine, an opium-derived narcotic similar to morphine but with much less risk of addiction. Codeine can be given on a regular basis for some months with little danger of dependence; however, tolerance does develop, which means the dose needs to be increased to continue providing relief.

Codeine was widely used in cough mixtures as it appears to have a special ability to stop the cough reflex. Since it is a narcotic, cough mixtures containing it can no longer be sold over the counter and have largely been replaced by formulas containing dextromethorpan which has no analgesic activity but is supposed to subdue the cough reflex.

The side effects of codeine are the same as other narcotics—constipation, nausea, and vomiting. Because of the low risk, superior pain-relieving qualities (to aspirin) and because it does not produce the euphoria, or "high," of stronger narcotics, codeine is a useful analgesic and is generally well liked by physicians.

Darvon (propoxyphene) is another analgesic about which there has been controversy. It is structurally related to methadone and claimed to be in the potency range of codeine with less risk of dependence. Dr. Michael Halberstam says,[4] "Darvon is stronger than aspirin. Not much, but stronger."

[4] *The Pills in Your Life,* Grosset & Dunlap, New York, 1972.

Dr. Halpern says, "Recent clinical trials have suggested that this product is difficult to distinguish from placebo in analgesic potency." As for addiction, he says that after giving large doses, discontinuance has produced withdrawal symptoms.

Percodan (oxycodone) resembles codeine, with similar or slightly better analgesic effect claimed. As with other narcotics, the side effects may include nausea, vomiting, and constipation. The manufacturer says, "The habit-forming potentialities of Percodan are somewhat less than morphine and somewhat greater than codeine. The same precautions should be observed as with other opiates."

Talwin (pentazocine) is a narcotic-like drug slightly stronger than codeine. The manufacturer claims that 50 mg. of Talwin is equivalent to 60 mg. of codeine. It is a weak narcotic antagonist, which means it has moderate action in blocking the effects of morphine or other narcotics, is not generally addictive itself, and usually produces fewer side effects. However, it may be erratic in that it works well with some patients and not at all with others. Side effects may include increased blood pressure, dizziness, nausea, and respiratory depression. At the pain clinic in Seattle, Talwin has been found useful, with a low incidence of addiction, and is considered an important addition to the analgesics.

STRONGLY ADDICTIVE DRUGS

There are many of these, the most important for analgesia are probably morphine, Demerol, and methadone.

Demerol (meperidine) is a synthetic narcotic, similar in many respects to morphine. It is a strong analgesic, but requires a dose of 50 to 100 mg. for the same effect as 10 mg. of morphine. It is addictive like morphine, but does not produce the same euphoria and so is not abused to the same extent as morphine or heroin. Like morphine, Demerol changes the patient's perception of his pain; he still feels it, but his anxiety is reduced and he is calmer and more comfortable about it. Like morphine, Demerol is constipating and may produce nausea and vomiting.

Dr. Halpern, in fact, thinks that the differences between morphine and the synthetic agents like it have been exaggerated. In comparable doses, he feels, the synthetics produce about the same euphoria and the same spectrum of side effects.

The Medical Letter, a publication which reports on drugs for physicians, distributed in December 1958 an article titled "Morphine versus Demerol." The conclusion reached was that the drug of choice for severe pain was still morphine, that Demerol was no more effective in relieving severe pain than morphine and did not cause less respiratory depression than morphine.

Again in August 1973, *The Medical Letter,* commenting on medication given the patient before anesthesia for surgery, was consistent in preferring morphine where there was pain. Other drugs used for preoperative pain include Talwin and Sublimaze (fentanyl), but again *The Medical Letter* saw no advantage over morphine.

Methadone is quite similar to morphine, so similar that it is popularly known for its use in withdrawing addicts from heroin. It is, however, much more than that.

"Methadone," says Dr. Halpern, "is nothing more than a synthetic opiate that has about the same potency as morphine, although it probably is not as good for all sorts of things as morphine is.

"No drug, no synthetic drug, has the ability to cover all of the bases that morphine does in full analgesic doses in people. And morphine is problematical because it has side effects and you don't give morphine to people who are going to get up and run around—you usually watch them in bed because of the cardiovascular hypotensive effects (lowered blood pressure), but morphine is still the best thing we have.

"There are lots of synthetics and you buy some advantages, such as duration of action or frequency or nonfrequency of certain side effects, but basically when you need full-blown analgesia, you turn back to morphine.

"Methadone is a nice drug for us to use in chronic pain patients because, in the patient who has tolerance, you get a beautiful long duration of action with methadone, which is why it's used on the street (for heroin addicts); you can cover a patient with it for thirty-six hours after an oral dose, provided he has tolerance.

"So the patients we see who are chronic pain patients, who were getting jagged medication every four hours—and by jagged medication I mean sharp changes in blood levels of the drug—have good coverage for awhile and then sit there and wait for the next medication, and then they have good coverage again.

You switch them over to methadone and give them a stable level and they stay at the same place for hours and hours and hours. Which means that they're not in pain, there's no alteration of state, and you can give the patient probably better coverage with that than you would with any other drug.

"As for their anxiety state—that's an interesting thing. When a patient comes to us they usually have high doses of a variety of different kinds of medication aboard. They are not only taking opiates, they are usually taking tranquilizers—minor tranquilizers like Librium or Valium—and barbiturates for sleep and things like that. All these drugs are usually short, intermediate-acting drugs and the patient cycles through them—it's incredible.

"They get very anxious between drug-taking times—they are actually in moderate withdrawal at these levels. So one of the things we do is to take away all their short-acting medication and substitute long-acting medications. And what that does immediately is to tell the patient that something has changed. Because all those periods of anxiety he used to incur during the afternoon before the nurse came in with his dose are gone. So obviously we must be doing something for him. We get a handle on his biological clock, and that changes his behavior.

"The other thing that we do very frequently is to take chronic pain patients for whom we do not see a clear-cut reason to continue medication and we simply detoxify them. And frequently enough the pain goes away as they become detoxified.

"In that particular situation the patient has probably been covertly requesting drugs by saying, "I hurt." *They* don't know this is going on. When you start to detoxify them of course, the whole game changes—the pain game changes—and pretty soon they realize they're not going to get more drugs by complaining about pain, so they don't talk about pain any more.

"We do a very slow detoxification. We decrease the dose and keep them in moderate withdrawal so that they are not at all uncomfortable. We tell them what we are doing. We get full consent. Full advice and consent. It's very difficult to do placebo games on people any more in terms of what the law says. And I just sit down at the bedside and say, 'Now look, we can't evaluate specifically what your pain problem is because you've got so much medicine aboard that you're impeding any diagnosis. If the physician presses you here, you don't feel anything, so he can't tell what's going on. Okay?'

"So they agree and you detoxify them. And as they start going down—most people go down very smoothly—in some cases the pain goes away. In other cases it doesn't go away and they're able to localize it and decide how much of what, and what treatments can be done because now the patient is describing something that is real."

Not every patient is willing to face the prospect of being without the drugs he has come to depend upon, and some will become anxious. This is recognized.

"You have to find different reasons to motivate people to bear with this. It's not an uncomfortable procedure. But of course if you've been laid back every four hours for the last fourteen years by a nice dose of something that makes you feel warm and pleasant, you get to look forward to it.

"One of the side effects of taking opiate medications is the fact that people become impotent. They have difficulties with their sex lives, and in many cases there are some severe problems between husbands and wives.

"We had one man coming in—he was the local motorcycle rider who had a polycystic kidney disease, with severe pain. He used to ride up to the outpatient window in his local dispensary and they'd shoot him full of junk and he'd ride off—it was incredible. He had a flap in his black motorcycle jacket and they used to inject—it was comical.

"Then we got him in the hospital and he was really on high medications of opiate and he was talking about the fact that he hadn't been able to make it with his wife for a long time. I said, 'If you give me five days, I'll give you a pass for the weekend. See how you like it.'

"So I detoxified him in the first five days, he went out over the weekend, came back with a broad smile, and I took him down to zero three days later. No problems.

"There was something he wanted, so we were able to do it. But you have to pay careful attention to the quantity and variety and essentially the frequency with which these drugs are used. Many people we see are out of the bounds of normal anxiety patients. There are many borderline psychotic if not frank psychotic patients.

"Some of these people use their drug to compensate for the psychiatric illness. They use their morphine or other opiate to do that. And you have to be very careful in these cases because once you get in and start playing the detoxification game they can do something really schizophrenic, so you have to be very careful to make sure that they're on the right medications, which should be antipsychotic drugs rather than the opiates."

Patients can be classified in dozens of different ways, but one way is to divide them into three main groups. First are those with acute pain, preoperative or emergency in nature, whose problem is medically fairly simple. Take care of the emergency and it's done.

Second are the otherwise normal people who, for some reason, have a chronic pain problem, but who are not anxious for neurotic reasons to hold on to it.

And third are the neurotic, the psychotic or near-psychotic, who bring along their psychological problems with their pain— "and all sorts of varieties and combinations in between. Drug use may be a primary problem; for example, the patient may be a frank drug-abuser. Or there may be a problem which confounds a clinician and calls for an absolutely legitimate drug use. You can tell after a while by the pattern and the frequency and the quantity of drug taken whether the patient is a drug-abuser or is just doing what his doctor told him to do.

"If the chronic pain patient has a condition that immobilizes him, you've got one sort of problem. If he has a condition that doesn't immobilize him, you've got a different situation. You then have someone who wants to be active, but is kept essentially incapacitated by the medication, and that's wrong.

"So what you've got to do is to give him the best coverage commensurate with the kind of activity level that he wants to maintain. Which means withdrawing him to a certain point and keeping him on enough medication or alternate techniques so that he can be active. There's no worry about keeping a patient on drugs indefinitely as long as the drugs are doing him no particular harm.

"Nor is addiction a particular harm, regardless of popular belief. Addiction is not a reason to take medication away from a patient.

"The terminal cancer patient [5] presents two different kinds of problems. A lady comes into the hospital and she's just awful-

[5] See Chapter 16.

looking. Her hair isn't combed, she's absolutely panicked, she's more anxious than you could ever believe, she knows she's going to die—what's her problem? Her problem is she's got so many things to do and the medication is keeping her down. She wants to go visit the grandchildren in Alaska before she dies. So what do you do for this woman?

"You detoxify her as much as possible. Two days into the detoxification and she's combing her hair and she's making plans. Halfway through the detoxification she's up and she's gone. She'll do the rest herself because she's got the time now and she wants to use it.

"Her pain? Pain wasn't her problem. Somebody was taking good care of her and giving her enough dope to slow her down. *That* was her problem.

"Another patient comes into the hospital and is totally incapacitated by the fear of dying. In which case you prescribe very high doses of medication and keep him snowed all the time.

"But you've got to do that with a full discussion with the patient and with the patient's family. And in a very sensitive way. You just can't take the responsibility to say, 'All right, I'm going to put you out of your misery.' You don't do that. You have to determine what the patient wants to do and how much discomfort—not pain, discomfort—the patient is willing to live with to get by."

Which brings us full circle back to the original question—what is pain? Is it as simple as Charlie Brown says: "Pain is when it hurts"?

"The meaning of that hurt is different with different people. I burned my hand, badly; it was [a] French-fried hand, that's what it was. And I looked at it and I figured, well, that's really going to hurt and what you have to do in a situation like this is, one, get the grease off, and two, occlude the air.

"So I went and made myself an occlusive pack with a pillow-case and some wadding, and then I went to the hospital and started to work on the hand. It hurt like mad.

"But the hurt was no concern to me at that particular time because I didn't have enough information about the extent of the injury to be worried, and I'm used to the clinical type. Somebody else might have been totally incapacitated by the pain and not be able to think and be totally disorganized by it.

"So people's responses to an injury which we call pain vary. You can't consider everybody's response to be equal. And you can't treat everybody the same way. You just can't do it.

"Sure the pain is there. You might say the patient has some sensory information which is discomforting. But his response to that information is the determining factor in how he will proceed."

All well and good. But shouldn't the doctor consider it a reasonable goal to remove the pain, to make the patient comfortable?

"I'm not sure those two things are incompatible, having pain and being comfortable. This is one of the things I've learned. It's a surprising thing to think about.

"The patient comes into the hospital and he's had nine operations on his back—which isn't uncommon. He has terrible pain. And he's afraid to move because he's likely to have more pain if he moves.

"The surgeon says, 'We're going to do it again. We'll operate again.' And the patient gets his hopes up and he goes through the operation and nothing happens.

"Now consider what happens when he comes into a place like this and we tell him, 'Now look, you've got enough scars on your back. No operation in the world is going to eliminate that condition. Now what you've got to do is to figure how you're going to be able to do things with that level of discomfort, if that's what you really want to do.' This is where Fordyce comes in." [6]

One might expect that this kind of pronouncement would throw the patient into a panic. He's going to be left alone with his pain.

"It doesn't throw him into a panic. Not necessarily. He's not going to be left alone with his pain. What he's going to be taught is how to live with his pain.

"If you can relieve pain with an analgesic drug and have it go away, that's nice. But after six weeks that doesn't work either. You can't count on medication to relieve chronic pain.

"And surgery isn't always the answer because even with surgery in many situations you can get a return of pain after six

[6] See Chapter 10.

months or so, although in others it's absolutely curative. So there is no formula.

"But with drugs, if the pain process goes on longer than six weeks or so and you're depending on the drug to alleviate the pain, you might as well forget it. It's not the addiction problem. But one of the problems with continued chronic medication is the factor of tolerance—you have to keep increasing the dose.

"Now when you get to high doses of opiate you buy a whole bunch of different kinds of problems. The idea is that within a six-week period you've run the patient up to about as high a dose as you're going to be able to, and if that doesn't keep the pain off, or if you don't have some other intervention ready to go, you might as well back off the drug because now you're going to start buying personality deficits and depression, you're going to change his outlook on life and constipate him and a lot of other things. You're going to make it difficult for him to go back and think about what the pain problem was when he started."

Since this discussion began with the assertion that the opiates do not kill pain but merely change the patient's perception of pain, it would appear logical that tranquilizers and similar psychotropic agents might also work. In fact, they do. By reducing anxiety, relieving depression, or altering psychotic behavior they do have an effect on pain. Used in combination with an analgesic they are more effective than when used alone, or when the analgesic is used alone. Properly chosen tranquilizers may have the effect of an additional 5 mg. of morphine in pain-relieving effect —which is a 50 percent improvement.

Some tranquilizers have their own addiction potential and long-term usage can lead to dependency. The result, as with the opiates, can be intensified emotional problems and an increase in pain. Then it becomes necessary to go through a detoxification process just as with the opiates. Withdrawal from tranquilizers, sedatives, or hypnotics can be achieved with phenobarbital which itself is then reduced by 10 to 15 percent a day.

It is a paradox that pain leads to the taking of drugs which leads to increasing the dose, which can lead to more pain and to behavior problems. But when the drug is then systematically withdrawn, the pain frequently improves as the patient comes out of his confusion and depression.

The doctor's dilemma is to understand that sometimes requests for pain drugs are genuinely for pain and sometimes they are ploys to support a drug addiction. In such cases an alternative must be found.

At the City of Hope National Medical Center, Dr. Crue supports a confidence in the psychotherapeutic drugs. "I wouldn't want to practice neurosurgery in the field of pain now without the newer pharmacological antidepressant drugs. Over the years I've used a lot of Merck's Triavil. It doesn't just help the psychotic depression, it helps the depressions that go along with chronic pain. The drugs like Trilafon and Elavil have really, in my opinion, revolutionized the treatment of things like post-herpetic neuralgia and atypical facial neuralgia, and we can get much better results than we ever could with any narcotics or analgesics in the past."

He has no major worry about sustained treatment with these drugs.

"A lot of our people are now using Pfizer's Sinequan for depression, and our psychiatrist here is testing it against Triavil to see if it works as well in chronic pain. We agree that the tricyclic effect isn't usually sudden, but if it's going to work it's rather dramatic, and takes place anywhere from a few days to a week or ten days. If it isn't going to work by the end of a couple of weeks, we don't use it. But if it does work we keep the patient on it almost indefinitely.

"I've had patients who have been on Triavil for six or eight years. Every once in a while they'll call up and they're depressed and they're hurting again. They will often say, 'Well, I was feeling so good I went on vacation and I stopped my Triavil.'

"It has a real effect. On a clinical, non-double-blind, noncontrol basis I'm convinced that some of these newer tricyclic compounds have revolutionized our treatment of some of these chronic pain cases." [7]

Comparisons of drug effects are difficult to make since pain

[7] Dr. Crue is here talking about straight clinical treatment of patients without control groups. A double-blind trial, standard in the pharmaceutical industry, divides patients into at least three groups. One group gets the drug under test, another gets a standard drug in the same field, the third gets a placebo or sugar pill without medical value. All pills are masked by code numbers and neither the doctor nor the patient knows which group is getting which medication or the placebo.

is so much a subjective experience. But many attempts have been made to assess pain levels using two criteria: "pain threshold," which refers to the minimal pain perceived, and "pain tolerance," which refers to the maximum pain which can be tolerated. The concept of pain thresholds is under strong fire from those who see the pain experience as a perceptive process. Two recent studies will convey the idea.

A double-blind study performed at the Queen's University of Belfast, Northern Ireland, was on drug effect in controlling pain in preoperative patients.[8] The conclusions reached in this test were that the subjective evaluation of pain, either by the patient or by an observer was in both cases sensitive and valid, assuming that, in fact, pain relief was what was being measured, not something else.

Drugs of the opium class may relieve pain by various mechanisms—raising the pain threshold, altering the patient's mood, or by putting him to sleep. To claim analgesia, the drug should actually relieve the pain, not produce stupefaction or euphoria. From the clinical standpoint the patient should be restored to a pain-free state rather than merely be blanketed by sedation or elevated into an unnatural elation.

The second study came out of the Department of Medicine and the Rheumatic Diseases Study Group of the New York University Medical Center.[9] This was the third of a series. The first had compared morphine, aspirin, and a placebo. The second had compared codeine and a placebo. The third compared codeine, aspirin, secobarbital, and a placebo. (Note: Codeine and aspirin are analgesics; secobarbital is a sedative of the central nervous system depressant type used mostly as a sleeping pill.)

In all three studies of this series, pain was produced experimentally in volunteers by two methods: applying an electric current to two fingers of the hand, or exposing the hand to cold pressor stimulation with ice water.

The two earlier studies had produced results which seemed to

8 William B. Loan, James D. Morrison, and John W. Dundee, "Evaluation of a Method for Assessing Potent Analgesics," *Clinical Pharmacology and Therapeutics,* Vol. 9, No. 6, November-December 1968, pp 765-76.

9 B. Berthold Wolff, Thomas G. Kantor, Murray E. Jarvik and Eugene Laska, "Responses of Experimental Pain to Analgesic Drugs," *Clinical Pharmacology and Therapeutics,* Vol. 10, No. 2, March-April 1969, pp. 217-28.

show that experimentally produced pain could be modified by morphine and codeine, while aspirin showed no significant effect. It should be noted that Beecher had questioned the validity of extrapolating results from laboratory-induced pain to the problems of naturally occurring real pain. The circumstances under which one or the other could occur changes the reactive components, and experimental pain is not the same as pain that occurs from illness or injury. Vital elements such as fear, apprehension, and worry are missing from a laboratory experiment.

Still, and with these reservations in mind, the Wolff studies suggest that pain *tolerance*—maximum pain—is more affected by analgesic drugs than pain *threshold*—minimum pain.

The drugs employed were codeine sulfate at 60 mg., secobarbital at 100 mg., aspirin one gram, and a placebo of milk sugar, all in identical-appearing capsules, coded and administered in a double-blind procedure.

Codeine produced the highest mean pain tolerance, with secobarbital next, and aspirin third. All three produced fairly close mean pain thresholds—their similarity bears out the conclusion that the effect was greater on pain tolerance than on pain threshold. Levels for the drugs in all the tests were higher than those for the placebo. It is significant, too, that there was a measurable effect from the placebo, which tells you something about the nature of drugs and their effect on the human nervous system, but tells you much more about the human nervous system and the importance of suggestion.

Chapter 9

NERVE BLOCKS AND NEUROSURGERY

The beneficial effects (of nerve block) outlast by hours, days and sometimes weeks the transient interruption of nerve impulses. It has been suggested that block of sensory input for several hours interrupts the self-sustaining activity of the neuron pools in the neuraxis, which apparently are responsible for some chronic pain states.

RICHARD G. BLACK, M.D.
JOHN J. BONICA, M.D.[1]

What to do then for the patient with unbearable pain who doesn't improve and cannot be kept on strong opiates indefinitely?

There are two more possibilities: nerve blocks and nerve surgery—cutting or destroying a section of the affected nerve fibers. We have been told that cutting the telephone lines doesn't always stop the messages. But sometimes it does, and under some conditions there is little else to do, for example, the cancer patient whose pain comes from a malignancy itself beyond surgery. In benign chronic pain, as Dr. Black and Dr. Bonica suggest, interrupting the pattern of uncontrolled repetitive neuron-firing

[1] "Analgesic Blocks," *Postgraduate Medicine*, Vol. 53, No. 6, May 1973, pp. 105-110.

may end its self-sustaining character and bring long-lasting relief. The pain doctors feel nerve blocks are worth trying, especially where there is a clear-cut choice between blocking and opiates.

Between surgery and blocks, the nerve block is the lesser extreme in its assault on the body. It is also not as final, particularly if an analgesic agent is used for temporary effect rather than a neurolytic agent like alcohol or phenol. If and when the effects of the block wear off, it can be repeated, and there is a worthwhile chance that the relief from pain may become permanent.

Injecting a local anesthetic into the area around a nerve temporarily suspends all messages, coming or going, from the central nervous system. The relief from pain brings several immediate benefits to the patient: an uplift in spirits and outlook, improved function of the involved limbs or muscles, better sleeping and eating, and the opportunity to begin physical therapy such as massage, heat, or traction, any of which would have been intolerable during the period of severe pain.

There is another function of nerve block. It can be used as a diagnostic tool to try to decide where and by what pathways the pain is coming, or as a prognostic device for a guess as to how a more permanent procedure might work, such as a block with a destructive agent like alcohol or surgery. These, however, are generally reserved for cases of inoperable cancer, or intractable conditions like trigeminal neuralgia, with its excruciating facial pain.

The temporary block gives the patient a chance to assess the side effects, what Dr. Crue calls "trading numbness for pain." The numb sensation may be almost as hard to live with as the pain, but this is always a subjective decision.

An interested observer of the initial nerve block may well be the neurosurgeon. From the temporary result he may draw conclusions about what to expect from the actual severing of the nerve. It remains at best an educated guess because a good response to nerve block does not insure success with a following operation. In fact, surgery is often not as effective in patients with benign chronic pain as it is with cancer patients.

"This," says Dr. John D. Loeser,[*] "may be due to the surgeon's

[*] Assistant Professor of Neurological Surgery; member, Pain Clinic, University of Washington Medical Center, Seattle, Washington.

failure to establish an accurate anatomic or pathologic diagnosis, or to comprehend fully the neural pathways involved in the transmission of pain, but a significant proportion of poor results seem to be related to failure to grasp the significance of the word 'pain,' and the role of pain behavior in the patient's environment." [2]

The surgeons too recognize the psychological content of pain and the conflicts of the chronic pain patient who might conceivably benefit more from other strategies than from surgery. So there is no rush to cut. Not everyone will benefit even from analgesic nerve block. Thorough evaluation of the patient and his medical problems must be done, and, says Dr. Black, the physician should take the time to become thoroughly acquainted with the patient, assess his personality, and establish mutual confidence.

Nearly a hundred years of experience with nerve block have produced a reasonably comprehensive guide to injection sites, techniques, and types of anesthetic for various pain conditions. Novocaine and its successors, Xylocaine, Nupercaine, and Marcaine, are all used locally, the first two being relatively short in duration of effect, the last two relatively long. A simple temporary condition, the type of muscle pain an athlete might suffer, could be relieved by injection of one of these anesthetics, plus a corticoid to reduce inflammation.

Receptors of the sympathetic nervous system can be blocked by injections at one of three critical sites. Somatic nerve blocks are used for neuralgia, and cranial nerve blocks for severe head pain. Spinal nerve block is used for pain in the back of the head and the neck, which can come from arthritis, or in young people from an injury such as whiplash.

Nearly all spinal nerves are mixed sensory and motor fibers and cannot be blocked without affecting use of the muscles. There are obviously limitations and disadvantages, the danger of complications, and no real assurance of beating the pain every time. For the most part, this is a hospital procedure requiring skilled professional backup help with resuscitative equipment on hand in case of severe reaction from the shots.

Blocks have been used for the pain of childbirth—the para-

[2] "Neurosurgical Relief of Chronic Pain," *Postgraduate Medicine,* Vol. 53, No. 6, May 1973, pp. 115-19.

cervical nerve is blocked with Marcaine and adrenaline during labor. In a trial reported by Kenneth Cooper, K. G. Gilroy, and D. J. Hurry, of Southlands Hospital in Sussex, England, 113 blocks were performed on 102 women. Pain relief was judged complete in 78, good in 20, and partial in 15. The average duration of effect was three hours and six minutes in all patients, an improvement over earlier trials using Xylocaine, which lasted only one to two hours.

Differential spinal block has also been used as a diagnostic device to trace the origin of low-back pain. One such experiment was reported by Brothers and Finlayson of the Department of Anesthesia, St. Michael's Hospital and the University of Toronto. Forty-eight patients with low-back pain were referred from the orthopedic or neurosurgical services. Forty had had previous surgery with temporary or no pain relief, and were suffering pain or incapacity out of proportion to the observed pathology.

Four types of block were performed: a sympathetic nerve block, a sensory nerve block, a motor nerve block and a placebo. Xylocaine was used for the actual blocks.

Patients who reported relief of pain after receiving the placebo, or conversely those who got no relief from full anesthesia, were judged to have no disease or organic reason for pain. Relief obtained from sympathetic or sensory blockade was judged to have an organic basis. Partial pain relief was considered of mixed origin—organic pain with psychological overtones. The differential block was useful in sorting out these causes and sources of the pain.

In the hands of an experienced practitioner, differential blocking can be a precise tool. Dr. Bonica points out in *The Management of Pain* that in treating facial neuralgia, differential diagnosis by nerve block can pinpoint whether it is the fifth, ninth, or tenth cranial nerve that is affected.

Where an abdominal pain is obscure enough to defy diagnosis, selective blocking can help differentiate between coronary disease, inflammation of pancreas or gallbladder, or a ruptured peptic ulcer. Similarly, paravertebral block can be used to differentiate between diseases of the chest and abdomen.

Nerve blocks are not innocuous, and are used only after conservative methods have failed to produce results. Even then, only selected cases will be likely to show success, and without care in selection, results may be poor.

All these cautions are doubled in the case of actual nerve surgery. The aim is to sever or destroy sections of the nerves carrying the pain messages, whether these be peripheral (nerves outside the spinal cord or brain) or central (in the spinal cord or brain).

Cutting a peripheral nerve is called a neurectomy, cutting into the central column is called a tractotomy. Neurectomy cuts a peripheral nerve in the hope that it will block just that part of the body from which the pain seems to emanate. The success rate is not very high for a number of reasons. Nerves overlap in their coverage, so that cutting one leaves other receptors still responding, or adjoining undamaged nerves may branch out to the denervated areas, or there may be other reasons.

To widen the affected area, the surgeon comes in closer to central to cut a bundle of sensory nerve fibers at the "root" where they converge to enter the central column or spinal cord. This is called a rhizotomy.

Cutting the sensory root of cranial nerves is an established procedure for severe pain of malignancies or for tic douloureux—facial neuralgia.

Dorsal rhizotomy, which cuts the nerve root where it enters the posterior side of the spinal column, is used for pain in the chest or abdominal wall. Dr. Loeser takes a dim view of this operation, believing it has many disadvantages. It is a major operation, frequently involving laminectomy, or removal of portions of a vertebra. Its influence on pain areas is restricted and it may alter pain patterns undesirably.

What seems like an even more critical procedure is regarded more favorably—this is cordotomy, or cutting a section of the white matter of the spinal cord itself, the anterolateral quadrant. It is a well-established operation for the relief of pain, especially since new techniques have been developed by which the surgeon probes through the skin instead of doing an open operation.

Cordotomy is supposed to provide a selective lessening of pain without loss of other functions, such as touch, or the risk of diminished motor control, which can happen when a mixed nerve is cut. However, the anesthesia may wear off after some years and the pain may return, at which time repeating the operation is ineffectual. For this reason, cordotomy too is used primarily for cancer patients in severe pain.

Cutting nerve tracts can be done in the brain stem—the medullary tractotomy is similar to the spinal cordotomy, and surgical lesions performed in the midbrain and thalamus are occasionally used for pain resistant to other measures. This is obviously critical and is done only when necessary by surgeons skilled in stereotactic surgery, a method of precise positioning of the surgical instrument from outside, without the necessity of making a large opening for direct observation.

Dr. Crue, of the City of Hope, has reported a refinement of the stereotactic technique using a bipolar electrode slim enough to be inserted in a standard 19-gauge needle. The needle is introduced through the foramen magnum, the opening in the occipital bone at the back of the head, which connects the vertebral canal and the cranial cavity. The bipolar electrode makes it possible to get signals back to verify the location of the nerve tract before a radiofrequency lesion is burned in the tract.[3]

This technique shows promise in accurately locating the target area. Patients with uncontrolled cancer have had significant relief from pain. Relief was not as consistent in trigeminal neuralgia, but there was some success, and as the technique is improved, better results may be obtained.

The ultimate, perhaps, in these surgical procedures is cingulumotomy—precisely positioned lesions made in the frontal lobe of the brain. There is a resemblance here to prefrontal lobotomy which has earned a bad name, but the destruction in cingulumotomy is narrower and more controlled, and there does not seem to be a danger of personality alteration. The effect is somewhat like that of the opiates—cingulumotomy does not raise the pain threshold but changes the patient's perception of pain.

It is obviously a very critical procedure and is only used to alleviate intense suffering when other techniques have not been successful.

The use of white noise as a masking device for pain has been

[3] B. L. Crue, E. J. A. Carregal, and A. Felsoory, "Percutaneous Stereotactic Radiofrequency Trigeminal Tractotomy with Neurophysiological Recordings," *Confinia Neurologica*, Vol. 34, No. 6, 1972, pp. 389-97.

mentioned (see page 22). Surgical techniques include an electrical kind of white noise. Low-voltage electrical stimulation is used to overload the large nerve fibers to block pain sensations coming up the small fibers, all in accord with the Melzack-Wall gate theory. It seems to work an impressive number of times.

One such device is called a dorsal column stimulator. It is surgically installed on the spine by removing a portion of a vertebra. Dr. C. Norman Shealy of the Pain Rehabilitation Center in La Crosse, Wisconsin, has done pioneering work with this and other forms of electrical stimulation, reporting on it at the International Symposium on Pain in May 1973 at the University of Washington School of Medicine.

Since 1967, Dr. Shealy said, his center has treated 1,500 patients with chronic pain by a variety of methods. About 25 percent of patients have shown a good response to external electrical stimulation, with partial relief for another 60 percent. Seventy-five patients have had dorsal column implants and another eighteen have had peripheral nerve implants. Overall, 20 percent of the patients have not been helped.

At Massachusetts General Hospital in Boston, Dr. William Sweet and Dr. James G. Wepsic have followed the progress of 138 patients who have had some form of electrical stimulation, either through the skin or by means of implanted electrodes under the skin, or near the posterior column of the spine. About a third of the patients followed for more than six months were said to have had good results—reduction of pain and resumption of normal activities with or without small doses of medication.

The transcutaneous stimulator, which applies an electrical current to the skin, is being used in Seattle, and another report on it came from the team of Dr. Howard L. Fields, Dr. John Adams, and Dr. Yoshio Hosobuchi at the University of California Medical Center in San Francisco. They found dramatic relief achieved in six out of eight patients with causalgia, a condition of chronic pain following an injury or burn. However, this relief was temporary, lasting somewhat over two hours after two minutes of stimulation.

Dr. Donlin M. Long of the University of Minnesota Hospitals, in Minneapolis, treated 500 patients with cutaneous electrical stimulation. The largest group of patients were eighty-nine with

low-back pain. The rest had a variety of problems, from degener-
ative osteoarthritis, phantom limb and facial pains, to spinal cord
injuries.

Of the entire group, 39 percent showed excellent relief with
pain more or less completely removed, and good results continuing with home use of the device. Of the rest, 28 percent showed
good results, and 33 percent were judged to be failures. Dr. Long
comments that the external stimulation appears to be a good way
of screening patients for the implantation of an electrical stimulator, and that the technique seems to have value in providing
relief for those seriously incapacitated by chronic pain.

The interest in electrical stimulation and other devices includes a recognition that surgery for the relief of pain can be
effective but has a considerable failure rate and is limited to certain conditions. Patients who have had multiple operations without relief are sometimes, in desperation, willing to try again, but
are not good choices for more surgery.

Where the underlying pathology does not account for the level
of pain suffered there is ample reason to avoid surgery and consider the part played by conditioning in pain behavior. For this,
an entirely new and different kind of therapy is needed.

Chapter 10

THE OPERANT PROGRAM

*The thing to keep in mind about chronic illness, including chronic
pain, is that you really have two problems. One is to reduce
sick-being and the other is to increase effective well-being. And those
aren't the same. If you do one it doesn't follow that you're
going to do the other.*

WILBERT E. FORDYCE, PH.D.[*]

At the time of her admission to Rehabilitation Medicine at the
University of Washington Medical Center, Mrs. M was thirty-
seven years old and had an eighteen-year history of back pain.

The pain, low in the back, had begun about a year after her
marriage and had become almost constant. Activity of any sort
made it worse, and she could not be active for more than twenty
minutes at a time before the increasing pain forced her to rest.
She was able to perform ordinary household tasks for a daily
total of less than two hours. The rest of the day was spent lying
down, reading, watching television, or sleeping.

Mrs. M had undergone four major surgical operations on her
back which included removal of a herniated disk and a spine

[*] Professor, Division of Clinical Psychology, Department of Rehabilitation
Medicine, University of Washington, School of Medicine, Seattle, Washington.

fusion. She was taking four or five addictive pain-relieving tablets a day.

Her physical examination and X-rays showed that her spine was stable at the site of the fusion, with no indication of neurologic problems.

Her consumption of analgesic tablets was irregular—she took them on demand, as she felt she needed them. This was the first thing changed. Medication was given on a regular time schedule whether Mrs. M felt she needed it or not. It was offered in a liquid form rather than the tablets she had been taking, with color and taste masked by cherry syrup or glyceryl guiacolate, a common ingredient of cough syrups.

The time between doses of medication was begun on a schedule to cover Mrs. M's pain, but it was gradually extended and the narcotic content slowly diminished. Meantime, she was placed in occupational therapy and not allowed to rest until she had finished the particular task she was doing. Her work in occupational therapy was geared to an increasing production schedule, so that her rest periods were moved further and further apart. She was also put into a walking program, with the distance walked gradually increasing.

A diary of Mrs. M's daily activities was begun. She had a daily fifteen-minute session with a psychologist to help her make graphs from her own records as a document of her progress, and her husband came in once a week to attend training sessions.

After thirteen days of the program, Mrs. M was working her full period of occupational therapy, just under two hours a day, without complaint or request for rest. At the end of seven weeks, she was walking almost a mile in the morning and again in the afternoon, at a speed double her previous pace. By the end of forty days her medication contained no narcotic at all, and a week later the doses were cut to once in four hours, with the night dose eliminated.

After eight weeks she was discharged on an outpatient basis and continued to be seen on a decreasing schedule. She bought a car for herself and became active and independent.

Why did it work? Nothing in the way of a surgical or medical miracle had been performed on Mrs. M. Yet she was better. As Dr. Fordyce might say, she had broken the pain habit, had "unlearned" her pain behavior.

There is a difference between pain that is a response to an intense noxious stimulus and chronic pain. "In chronic pain," Dr. Fordyce says, "the responses occur over long periods of time, thereby affording an opportunity for learned behavior. A patient intentionally or involuntarily signals to those around him that he has pain by using a set of actions termed operants. For example, a patient may describe his pain, walk and move in a guarded manner, grimace, ask for medication, call his physician for assistance, or decide that he will stay in bed." [1]

These behaviors are what B. F. Skinner* has called operants—behavior controlled by the consequences of what follows.

In trying to conceptualize pain problems, psychologists regard pain as a set of responses, as something the patient is *doing*. "Stated another way," says Dr. Fordyce, "the patient must engage in some behavior identified by observers as indicative of pain, that is, he must engage in pain behavior."

This would include doing nothing—he can sit still and concentrate on his hurt—that too is pain behavior.

The pain doctor begins with the premise that the pain may be caused by a pathogenic factor. Is there injury or disease present? His first effort, therefore, is to try to identify the suspected underlying pathology. If it can be discovered, treatment will be directed toward removing or relieving it and, hopefully, with it the pain. If no pathology can be discovered, or the pathology which is found appears minor in comparison with the amount of pain it seems to be producing, this suggests the presence of another set of pathogenic factors involving emotional or personality problems. There are a variety of terms to describe these: psychogenic pain, hysteria, conversion reaction or somatic reaction in which unacceptable unconscious impulses are converted into bodily symptoms.

This is not to say, nor is it fair to the patient to assume, that

---

[1] "An Operant Conditioning Method for Managing Chronic Pain," *Postgraduate Medicine,* May 1973, Vol. 53, No. 6, pp. 123-28.

* Harvard psychologist. Skinner has garnered bouquets and brick-bats for his best-known book, *Beyond Freedom and Dignity,* which expounds his operant theory that "desirable" behavior is rewarded in many ways. Objections centered around the definition of the word "desirable," with critics showing alarm at the prospect of a controlled society. Yet the application of operant theory to pain control is a natural one and less vulnerable to charges of a 1984 mentality.

merely because there is little or no pathology apparent his pain is due entirely to a personality disorder. Even where personality problems do exist, therapy aimed only at these problems does not do much to relieve the pain. Psychotherapy has a low rate of success in dealing with chronic pain. Anyone, with or without a personality problem, can learn the pain habit because such learning is inherent in conditions which reward pain behavior.

Presume that the original pain began with some sort of pathological stimulus, injury, or illness. There is a reason, as Dr. Crue has said, for the pain appearing in the exact way and the exact place that it does. Now consider that the conditions under which a particular individual lived had the effect of reinforcing pain-behavior and punishing well-behavior.

We have had one example of the wife with a tepid marriage who finds that her pain wins solicitude from an otherwise indifferent husband. Another might be the man who hates his job and gets some relief by acquiring an ulcer, which wins him preferential treatment from his boss, his friends, and his wife. Dr. Fordyce supplies the case of the laborer with chronic back pain whose ache is increased when he works and diminished when he rests. If he is allowed to rest when he complains of pain, rest itself becomes a reinforcer of pain by *rewarding* pain-behavior. Even though his back pain sprang from a wholly legitimate injury, the environmental stimuli continue to strengthen this operant behavior.

If it were possible to follow a pain patient at every moment and record that his pain-behavior was followed by this sort of reinforcing consequence, but that his *failure* to complain—his well-behavior—was ignored, as it quite normally would be, it is entirely possible that the individual would be urged in the direction of showing more pain-behavior and less well-behavior even though the original pathogenic factor may have disappeared.

Medication can be a reinforcing agent. It is common in treating pain for the physician to prescribe medication "p.r.n."—or "take as needed." The prescription then becomes an operant, since taking it or not taking it is contingent upon the presence or absence of pain. Thus the drug itself can reinforce the patient's habit of asking for medication and the frequency with which he asks. And it may help to develop dependence and addiction.

The pain habit can even be strengthened by faulty application of physical therapy. For example, exercises may be prescribed for the patient with low-back pain, with instructions to stop when pain begins, or to continue until the pain becomes intolerable.

In either case, a sequence of three distinct steps is set up: work, pain, rest. It is obvious that rest becomes a consequence of the appearance of pain. So, whether the patient realizes it or not— and usually he does not, rest becomes a reinforcer of pain-behavior. In short, says Dr. Fordyce, this creates the same kind of reinforcement as taking medication on demand; both may strengthen pain-behavior.

The operant conditioning program at Seattle attempts to deal with these environmental reinforcers by changing the pattern. "When an operant is followed by a negative consequence such as criticism or loss of valued rewards, that behavior is likely to occur less frequently in the future or decrease in strength, and behavior designed to remove the negative consequence or avoid it is likely to increase. When a behavior is followed by neither positive nor negative consequences, the behavior will tend to decrease in frequency, a process called extinction. These behavior-consequence relationships are basic elements of operant conditioning." [2]

As best it can, the pain clinic arrives at a decision as to what the problem is and what might be done about it. Its function is diagnostic. The patient then goes for treatment to any of a number of programs relating to the pain clinic, of which the operant program is one. Dr. Fordyce is on the staff of the pain clinic, but his primary activity is in rehabilitation medicine. His operant program takes perhaps one out of three patients from the pain clinic output. Others may go to neurosurgery, orthopedics, or anesthesiology for blocks.

"Any time a pain problem has lasted more than four to six months we would expect almost always there would be an element of learning that takes place. Habituation or learning. Now how much? It's going to vary enormously. The patients we see, when it's something other than arthritis or cancer or something like that, have a significant amount of it. We don't always feel there is something we can do about it. But if we think we can, we program basically rest, attention, and medication in a systematic

[2] Wilbert E. Fordyce et al., "Operant Conditioning in the Treatment of Chronic Pain," *Archives of Physical Medicine and Rehabilitation*, Vol. 54, No. 9, September 1973, pp. 399-408.

way consistent with operant conditioning or contingency management principles. The thing to keep in mind about chronic illness, including chronic pain, is that you really have two problems. One is to reduce sick-being, and the other is to increase effective well-being. And those aren't the same. If you do one, it doesn't follow that you're going to do the other.

"So that in our experience, with the people we select for the operant program, and we do select them, this is not a random sample of pain patients. For those we select it is relatively easy to reduce pain-behavior.

"It's not tough at all to get people off medication, to get their activity level up, and they don't complain as much about pain and they move around and do all sorts of things. But to keep it going, to get them involved in effective well-behavior so they can maintain their treatment gains is much more difficult.

"We tell a story, a true story, and I think it makes the point as well as anything I know, although it happens to relate to obesity rather than to pain. These behavioral systems can be used with obesity and lots of other conditions.

"One of our residents in a medical specialty who was chronically obese, about six feet two inches and 275 pounds, came to us and asked, 'Would you work with me, using your process?'

"So we set him up with a kind of do-it-yourself kit so to speak, which he used over seven or eight months. One Saturday I came into the hospital and went down to the cafeteria for a cup of coffee and there he was. I asked, 'How's it going?'

"He said, 'I reached my target weight last week. I want to tell you what happened. For the first time I felt that I was no longer ashamed to be seen on the diving board in a swimming suit. So I headed over to the men's gym, which is a couple of blocks over this way, and on the way over, I suddenly realized that I don't know how to dive.'

"And that's the way it is with chronically ill people. They've been on the sidelines so long that there are major gaps in their well-behavior repertoire. *They don't know how to be well.*

"So the system has got to do two things. It's got to reduce pain-behavior, but it's also got to increase effective well-behavior. And if you do one without the other you're not helping the patient. Reducing pain-behavior within the limits of our selectivity—that's pretty easy. The tough part is shaping an effective well-behavior. And that's the major weakness of our program. We're trying to strengthen it as much as we can, but that's tough to do.

"We just took in a lady from the East Coast and I'll be very much surprised if we can't decrease her pain. She may be one of the easiest patients we ever had. But what will she do then? If her pain is a response to some lack or imagined lack, how do we control that?

"Of course we have part of her family out here and we'll work with them. We won't accept a patient in the program unless the spouse participates. And we train the family, literally train them, to be selectively responsive to sick- and well-behavior.

"There is no element in this program that we do not describe in great detail to the patient and the family before we ever begin. We tell them everything. There are no secrets. This is not a Machiavellian manipulation-behind-the-scenes sort of thing. We tell them ahead of time what we are going to do and how we are going to do it. That will include people being selectively responsive to sick- and well-being. If your husband is here, or a daughter-in-law is here, we'll work with them, train them in how to do this.

"Now they are going to have to convey that back to the East Coast, to bring along the rest of the family. Of course there's more to it than just getting the family involved. That lady needs herself to become effectively involved in things that turn her on. And that's going to be a lot tougher to do. She's a very lonely lady." And, of course, in that one remark, Dr. Fordyce put his finger on one cause of pain in our society.

The goal then, in operant conditioning, is to identify the elements in the patient's environment which reinforce his pain-behavior and see what can be done about removing them. Throughout, Dr. Fordyce talks about pain-behavior rather than pain. This is significant, not incidental. It is at once the strength of the operant conditioning program, the thing that makes it work, and at the same time its vulnerable point, as we shall see.

Two other things need to be done. Medication has to be reduced and eventually eliminated, and physical activity must be increased. The first two refer to reducing sick-being, the last to increasing well-being.

The medication routine begins by placing the patient on a p.r.n.—take as needed—basis for two to four days. This is done so the attendants, a nurse if the patient is hospitalized, otherwise a member of the family, can make an accurate record of the amount taken and the times the patient asks for it. A record of physical activity is also kept. A base line for medication is now established, setting the limits within which the patient feels comfortable.

The next step is setting up the "pain cocktail." This is the pain medication in a liquid form, with color and taste hidden by a flavor vehicle such as cherry syrup. The dose and frequency are arranged to match the base line already established.

The big difference is that the medication is no longer given on a demand basis. It is given at regular fixed intervals around the clock, whether the patient wants it or not. In fact, the interval between doses is less than the interval normally established by the patient on his p.r.n. schedule. If the patient had averaged five or six hours between doses, cocktail time would come up every four hours on the new program.

The reason for this is that the pain cocktail does not become a positive reinforcer because it is not presented as a response to pain. Given when no pain is present, it is somehow no longer so closely associated in the patient's mind with the resumption of his pain.

Once this new pattern is established, the actual medication in the pain cocktail is gradually decreased. The patient (although he has been told about it) does not know exactly when this occurs because the flavor and color vehicle obscures any clues he might have as to the contents. Experience at the pain clinic has shown that a gradual decrease over a period of seven to eight weeks is slow enough to avoid withdrawal symptoms and give the patient's body a chance to adjust to the absence of the narcotic.

Although Dr. Halpern has found that frequently this procedure alone seems to work, in that the pain does not return, Dr. Fordyce does not let it go at that. He has been watching the patient's life-style for those reinforcers, those relationships between habits and pain, and conversely, the lack of reinforcers for well-behavior. A refusal to get out of bed, to engage in any interesting activities—these are obviously negative reinforcers.

Next, having identified the pain reinforcers which must be eliminated, and decided upon the behavior which must be increased, he must decide on a program to encourage the proper responses.

One thing he avoids is expressions of sympathy and much attention. These are powerful reinforcers of chronic pain-behavior. Not only does the pain doctor avoid these himself, he trains the patient's family to rigorously ignore complaints of pain or discomfort and to check any impulse to compassionate attention in spite of complaints. When attention is paid to the patient it is not for pain complaints, but when the patient is pushing himself into some kind of activity and particularly when he is raising the level of his activity. "In this way," says Dr. Fordyce, "pain-behavior receives a minimum of social reinforcement and activity receives a maximum of reinforcement."

A fine line has to be drawn between punishing a patient and promoting activity. To do this, the program rewards the patient with rest and attention, and praise when he makes progress.

Physical activity is encouraged in spite of complaints about pain. Here, too, as in the pain cocktail element, the procedure is the reverse of what would be expected. Working to tolerance actually increases pain-behavior. The alternative is working to quota.

Once again, the first step is to let the patient do what he feels he can do and so set a base line for his tolerance. Given an exercise to do, he performs it until the pain begins, or he becomes tired.

If he says he is always in pain, or any activity immediately brings on the pain, he is asked to continue to the point where the work sharply increases the level of pain, or he becomes very tired. This trial is done several times and, just as for his medication, sets a base line for effort.

Out of this a quota for exercise is established. Again, like the doses of medicine, the quota is conservative—at or below the lowest line of his recorded trials. This permits him to do a quota without exhaustion or intolerable pain knocking him out of the running before he has completed it. His sequence now becomes work—rest; not work—pain—rest. Thus rest, still a reinforcer, is dependent upon completing his work, not upon the appearance of pain. Rest becomes a reinforcer of completed activity rather than pain-behavior.

A few days of this and the quota can gradually be increased.

In not too long a time it passes the original tolerance limit, as seen in the case of Mrs. M. The record she kept, which is charted in a graph form, shows her and her family an immediate pictorial record of improvement and becomes itself a reinforcer of well-behavior.

The last link in the chain is the patient's home environment. Assuming he has made progress in rehabilitation, the medication has been eliminated, the physical activity increased, the complaints of pain diminished, the well-being strongly reinforced —what happens when he goes home? He falls back into an environment which repeats the conditions leading to the original problem—all the reinforcements of pain and the negative enforcers of activity.

This is the critical point, and it is for this that the family has been trained. They must cooperate seriously and fully to change the environment and keep it changed, otherwise the gains made in the rehabilitation clinic will fairly quickly be wiped out.

In most cases the patient's spouse was asked to come in for twice-a-week training sessions. Patients in the rehabilitation center receive a minimum of four weeks and a maximum of twelve weeks of treatment. After discharge they may have needed no outpatient follow-up, some have required additional treatment as long as twenty-four weeks.

The pain-behavior, reduced or extinguished, covered a variety of displays. Moaning, gasping, complaining verbally, grimacing or gesturing, walking as though on eggs, stopping activity to sit down or lie down because of pain and, of course, taking drugs.

The well-behavior activity increased, yet it differed with the individual patient. It included walking, working in the hospital or the university, or occupational therapy, which might mean weaving or operating a hand-printing press.

Training the patient's spouse meant educating him or her to identify and understand pain behavior and its consequences, as well as to identify properly well-behavior and its consequences, and to respond with the appropriate reaction to each type of behavior. To do this properly was to provide the patient with reinforcement of well-behavior while avoiding reinforcement of pain-behavior.

To lubricate the patient's eventual return to a work environment, where this was required, the in-hospital work assignment was something reasonably similar, such as a job in the hospital or university. If work was not the eventual goal, as in the case of a housewife, but a return to social activities, these contacts, with the help of the spouse, were gradually increased during the weeks of treatment.

Follow-up of discharged patients is something of a difficulty since many of them came long distances to the clinic. There are neither funds nor manpower for a face-to-face interview of patients scattered widely over the country. Dr. Fordyce compromised on a questionnaire. The average interval between the time of discharge and the follow-up questionnaire was twenty-two months.

One group of patients was asked to rate themselves on a 10-point scale as to (1) the pain they had when they first came to the clinic, and (2) the current pain at the time of receiving the questionnaire. Zero meant no pain at all, while 10 meant maximum pain.

Average ratings of pain intensity showed 8.57 at time of admission and 6.03 at time of discharge. At the time of the follow-up, average pain was 6.17. (There was a plus or minus factor in each number which we have dropped for simplicity.)

Obviously there was still a claim of considerable pain, although the improvement is real and the increase since discharge is small.

The patients were also asked to rate on the same 10-point scale the degree to which pain interfered with their activities. The average ratings now were: at admission 7.76; at discharge 4.83, and at follow-up 5.00. These figures showed a considerable improvement.

Finally they were asked to show the number of hours spent lying down or being up during the normal day—7:00 A.M. to 10:00 P.M. The returns showed an average uptime of 10.27 hours at admission time and 12.55 hours at follow-up time.

It seems fairly evident that the patients showed reduction in pain, but still claimed to have a considerable amount of pain. Yet they were more active than before and less complaining. In short, they had learned to live with their pain, even where it could not be eliminated. "It could be argued," Dr. Fordyce said, "that the pain was the same and the change was only in verbal behavior in response to the withdrawal of social reinforcers to verbal complaints of pain."

The still unresolved question is—what is pain? Is it a neuro-physiological phenomenon and a set of responses, or is it the responses themselves? It sounds like the old riddle: if a tree in the forest falls and no one is there to hear it, is there a sound?

Psychiatrist Donald Kornfeld, speaking at a panel session on pain at the 1973 annual meeting of the American Medical Association, said of the operant program that it was "treating the behavior, not the pain."

To which Dr. Crue is inclined to agree. "You get the patients so mad at the nurses that they've *got* to walk that extra step. If they walked ten steps the first day they walk twelve steps the second day and fifteen steps the third day so they can have TV that night. And by the end of six weeks they're off medication and walking one hundred steps. They came in walking ten steps and now they walk one hundred steps—that's a tenfold increase and there's every right to call this success.

"There's only one thing. The majority of patients will say 'I hurt as much as I ever did.' The patient isn't cured of his pain, he can just walk ten times as far."

Dr. Fordyce would disagree. What we say and what we do are not the same thing. He relates this story to make the point. Suppose you are treating a lady who dislikes snakes intensely. You have a snake in a basket and you ask her to take it out. She shudders and says she can't do it. Then you go through a program of desensitizing her to snakes and you get her to handle them in a controlled manner. After the desensitization program, you bring in the snake in its basket and ask her again to take it out. She does so without hesitation, without any grimace of distaste or any other visible symptom. This is the behavior you can see.

Then you ask her, "How do you like snakes now?"

She promptly says, "They're horrible—I can't touch them!"

So people can report one thing and do another. The point is, Dr. Fordyce says, that if someone says he has pain, but is learning to live with it, does he really have pain? He is reporting pain, but his actions say he does not have pain.

If he goes back to work and functions in spite of the pain he says he still has, is he better off? Is society better off?

Dr. Fordyce thinks both are. He believes the learning factor is a powerful element in chronic pain. His instructions to the incoming patient, a six-page, simply multigraphed paper, explains this and answers some of the more common questions which might be asked.

"Our knowledge about pain, what it is and what influences it," the paper says, "has changed a lot in recent years."

Briefly, one of these changes is that behavioral science has discovered that body processes can be influenced by conditioning or learning. It had been assumed that the only way to change basic processes inside the body was by surgery or medication. But not all people are helped by these methods and require something else to make the change.

"We usually think of learning as something we decide to do or not to do as the case may be. Actually, that is not the way it is. Learning is automatic—if the conditions for learning are right. If conditions for learning are right, we will learn whether we want to or not. If conditions for learning are not right, we will not learn, no matter how much we want to. Learning is not something you can turn on or off. All you can really turn on or off is whether or not you get into situations in which learning can occur."

Essentially this is the principle which controls the learning of pain. If conditions are right, the body learns pain, whether the person wants to or not.

The paper describes to the patient the proposed program of work, exercise, rest, and therapy, makes the point that since no two people are exactly alike, the individual program will vary as the situation requires. Then it takes up questions the patient may have in mind:

Q: Do you think my pain is imaginary—"just in my head?"

A: No. It is a mistake to think that pain is either "real," that is, organic or physical, or "imaginary," that is, psychogenic, hysterical, or hypochondriacal. Pain is a body process which starts with some form of tissue damage. If that damage persists long enough and conditions for learning have been such as to permit or cause learning or conditioning to occur, the pain may come under control of learning factors. Even if the tissue damage has been reduced or eliminated, the pain may continue as learned or operant pain. When that happens, the patient is no more capable of turning off the pain bell than he is of stopping his heartbeat.

Q: If I go through the operant program, will my pain be cured?

A: Probably not totally. If, after our evaluation, we feel the program is likely to be of help to you, you have a very good chance by the end of the program of (1) having a great increase in activity without pain, weakness, or fatigue being the major limiting factors; (2) if you take much pain medication, of being able to get along with little or no pain medication; and (3) of feeling significantly less pain than you did at the outset, with the amount of pain continuing to diminish gradually during the months after the program.

Q: Is the operant program just a way of teaching me to live with my pain?

A: No. It is probably true that in some cases the program works that way, too. Mainly, however, the operant program takes dead aim at the pain and works to reduce it.

Q: What happens if my pain doesn't get better?

A: We hope that working together, you and your family and we can significantly reduce your pain. Even if our gains are modest, it is almost always the case that we can help you both to reduce the amount of medication you need and want, and to increase your activity level so that you can do a lot more of the things you want to do without the pain interfering.

Q: Is the operant program a form of psychotherapy or psychiatric treatment?

A: No. The operant program for chronic pain is a form of treatment aimed at physical restoration.

Clearly enough, the operant program is not intended to displace other methods aimed directly at the physical causes of pain. It is used only when such other methods have been unable to help, and as a result the patient evaluation shows the existence of learned pain behavior. In such cases it is entirely logical to go to work on the behavior. In essence, what else is there to do?

Under one name or another, the operant program idea is spreading. At the University of Minnesota Hospital it is called "behavior modification." Dr. Theodore M. Cole, the hospital's specialist in physical medicine and rehabilitation, believes it works.

He says, "First of all, it is only natural to want to get rid of pain. In effect we're almost telling the person we aren't going to cure the pain. But we have found that as a patient conditions himself to our therapy, the pain does seem to diminish, or it may even vanish completely." [3]

So far there are no universal, infallible panaceas. But whatever does work, in whatever measure, deserves all the attention it can get.

[3] Michael W. Fedo, "Can You Will Away Pain?," *Family Health*, Vol. 4, No. 10, October 1972, pp. 32, 40-42.

Chapter 11

PAIN GAMES AND ALTERNATIVES

Patients in chronic pain engage in a variety of manipulative transactions with doctors. This applies both to those whose pain is primarily psychogenic and those whose pain is primarily somatogenic; the effect of chronic pain is to make formerly emotionally sturdy persons into neurotic manipulators.

RICHARD A. STERNBACH, PH.D.*

The uses of pain are many, and for some people they offer advantages apparently worth the distress and disability which must be endured. Pain can be a form of communication. It establishes a clear identity, even if it is the identity of an invalid. And, most important, it is a means for manipulating and controlling other people in a game of painmanship.

In his perceptive book, *Games People Play,*[1] Dr. Eric Berne described some of these transactions between doctors and patients. The game of "Ain't It Awful?" came in several variations,

* Adjunct Associate Professor of Psychiatry, School of Medicine, University of California, San Diego, and Veterans' Administration Hospital, San Diego, California.
[1] Grove Press, New York, 1964.

but its most dramatic form was reserved for the polysurgery addicts.

These were the people who went from doctor to doctor demanding surgery, rejecting contrary medical advice until they found a surgeon who would oblige. The operation fulfilled a need for self-mutilation, the hospitalization presented an opportunity to escape social intimacies and responsibilities. And afterward came the quintessence of the game, the telling and retelling with lingering details of the horrors endured to evoke awed sympathy from listeners.

This was the major payoff. "Ain't It Awful?" provided rewards derived from the satisfaction of contemplating one's own disasters and gaining status from the resulting notoriety.

Satisfactions can also be had from a game of "Wooden Leg," the essence of which is, "What can you expect from a man with a wooden leg?" Transpose this to the pain patient and you have, "How do you expect me to do anything when I am in such pain?"

Both games spell a cop-out and this is crippling enough. But, as Dr. Berne describes it, the ramifications of the game go beyond the patient. His family and friends may have their own game plans which can include, "I'm Only Trying to Help You," a game which provides various satisfactions but depends basically upon maintaining the patient in dependence upon the "helper." The rule of the game is, "I'm only trying to help you (so long as you don't get better)."

In some cases the therapist may run into outright opposition from relatives if they see the patient beginning to make progress. Says Dr. Berne, "All the people who were playing 'I'm Only Trying to Help You' are threatened by the impending disruption of the game if the patient shows signs of striking out on his own, and sometimes they use almost incredible measures to terminate the treatment."

Just north of San Diego, California, is a Veterans' Administration Hospital, a massive concrete structure atop a windswept hill. The hospital has a pain unit under the joint direction of Dr. Jerry H. Greenhoot, an Assistant Professor of Neurosurgery, and Dr. Richard A. Sternbach, a psychologist. A veterans' hospital encloses patients who surely have legitimate cause for pain. Yet this pain unit experience parallels that of the Seattle Pain Clinic in that they have found that patients with persistent chronic pain, no matter what the cause (including battle-caused wounds), develop "significant and persistent psychological problems."

"We have found," say Drs. Greenhoot and Sternbach, "that many of these patients cannot be categorized conveniently. Their problems do not respond to standard psychotherapeutic approaches. However, without the resolution of these problems, appropriate and well-planned neurosurgical intervention often fails to provide the expected rehabilitation. The patients either do not gain adequate pain relief, or following relief of pain they remain so miserable that they do not return to adequate social function.

"We have learned that the only adequate measure of success or failure of pain relief is the patient's behavior. A patient who has no pain, but who does not function adequately, has had a 'bad' result, while another with complaints of pain, but who lives well, has been rehabilitated." [2]

These findings parallel those of Dr. Fordyce, and part of the procedure of the San Diego Pain Unit follows lines essentially the same as the operant program at Seattle. But Dr. Sternbach's particular contribution has been his close study of painmanship—the games patients play—and the reaction of relatives, friends, and doctors.

"By virtue of disease or injury or emotional conflict," says Dr. Sternbach, "a person experiences continued pain and gradually comes to think of himself as a chronic invalid and suffering person." [3]

This becomes his new identity and the base line from which he launches the games needed to protect that identity. Conflict is inherent here because everyone wishes to be free of pain, yet the game is designed to prevent change, and the patient will fight to preserve this life-style based on pain.

In Berne's terms, a transaction is a unit of social intercourse, an exchange between two or more people. A game is a series of transactions with an ulterior motive leading to a preselected outcome. Every game, says Berne, is basically dishonest, and the

[2] "Conjoint Treatment of Chronic Pain," *International Symposium on Pain,* ed. Dr. John J. Bonica, Advances in Neurology, Vol. 4, Raven Press, New York, 1974.

[3] "Varieties of Pain Games," *International Symposium on Pain.*

outcome is deliberately dramatic. A typical first transaction between doctor and pain patient may go something like this:

PATIENT: Doctor, I'm in terrible pain. Help me. (I'll bet you can't.)
DOCTOR: I'm sure we can help you.
PATIENT: (That's what you think.)

The doctor prescribes, the patient submits, and there is little
or no relief. Consultants are summoned, the procedures are
changed, the patient goes through more rituals. There is still no
relief. The doctor admits bafflement. The next transaction occurs
with the patient asking:

PATIENT: What's wrong with me, doctor? (I told you you couldn't
cure me.)
DOCTOR: I don't know. I don't see any reason for so much pain.
PATIENT: (You quack. Where do I find a real doctor?)
DOCTOR: (You're a crock. It's all in your head.)

First game to the patient. For him it might have been a game
of "Gotcha!" He has maneuvered the doctor into an admission of
failure, which is the object of the game. Or it could have been
"Why Does This Always Happen to Me?", if he is full of self-pity,
confirming his identity as an incurable invalid.

He has, in either case, vindicated his status as a sufferer and
has shown the world that his illness is unique, that it cannot be
diagnosed or relieved. He has successfully fended off any move
to make him responsible for his own life, he has reaffirmed his
helplessness and his need to be taken care of and protected.

For some, the roots of this behavior may go back to early
transactions between parent and child. The child attempts to
excuse some misbehavior with the plea, "I don't feel good."

To which the angry parent responds, "I'll wallop you and you'll
feel that pretty good."

Punishment becomes justification for misbehavior and the pattern for masochism is set up and reinforced in ensuing transactions. The child recognizes punishment as a sign the parent is
concerned. Ignoring him would be worse than punishment.

CHILD: Hit me so I'll know you care about me. (But don't think I'm
going to change.)
PARENT: You'll change all right, or I'll beat you until you do.

This is a parallel to the transaction between the patient and the pain doctor.

PATIENT: I'm in pain. Help me. (But you can't.)
DOCTOR: Do as I say and I'll help you.

It is not at all necessary, Dr. Sternbach says, for the patient to have fashioned this model in childhood. An adult can learn it easily enough in two common steps: (1) acquiring severe chronic pain (through illness, injury, or emotional deprivation), and (2) reinforcing his pain behavior through operant conditioning. Successful reinforcement establishes the pain habit and launches a career as a professional pain patient.

"The life-style will continue," says Dr. Sternbach, "until there are no more payoffs, and satisfactory alternatives are offered."

Obviously the goals of the professional pain patient and those of the doctor are diametrically opposed to each other. The doctor's self-image is that of a healer; his role is to diagnose expertly and to relieve the patient's suffering. The patient is geared to resist any attempt at real cure. Should the doctor fail, there is strong compulsion to protect his self-image by labeling the patient a crock and getting rid of him by referring him to another specialty.

The patient meanwhile uses the doctor as a pawn in his game of "Wooden Leg." Who can expect him to get well when the doctors are unable to figure out what is causing his pain?

The professional pain patient can be identified by the barely concealed satisfaction with which he accepts the doctor's admission of failure to help him. Far from being depressed by it, his attitude, however concealed, is very much, "I knew it," with the larger issue of his pain buried under his victory in gamesmanship.

There are many varieties of pain games. Some patients confine themselves to one type, others are skilled in several. A good player can almost invariably beat the average doctor who is not generally prepared for this and may not recognize for some time that he is being used.

The fraudulent pain patient plays the game not for status but for money. This is the patient who creates injury or illness for insurance, workman's compensation, welfare or other payoffs. Obviously there is a gray area here, some patients are not outright frauds, but the compensation payments are a form of operant reward which reinforce their disabilities on a subconscious, not consciously ulterior level.

For our purposes we can disregard the outright fraud. We are here concerned with the patient who hurts genuinely, even though sometimes the line is hard to draw between the fraud and the conditioned patient.

Dr. William R. Halliday is Chief Medical Consultant for the State of Washington's Department of Labor and Industry. This department has been forward-looking in establishing a work-man's compensation rehabilitation program with Kenneth V. Settle as director. In a clinic setting, the rehabilitation program works to restore injured people to independent functioning in their lives.

"We no longer use such terms as 'conscious' or 'unconscious,'" Dr. Halliday says. "These are people who in many ways find themselves inadequate under certain circumstances and therefore develop pain behavior, or the disability process."

The injured workman, like the professional pain patient, claims to be eager to return to work, but finds multiple excuses for post-poning it. The tip-off to the professional pain patient, says Dr. Sternbach, is his refusal to consider any kind of work except what he had been doing and refusing anything which might be con-sidered stepping down to a lower level. An injured telephone lineman may be barred from climbing poles again, but how do you interpret his rigid refusal to accept a ground job—pride or malingering?

"Our approach in the workman's rehabilitation clinic," says Director Settle, "is through the use of medical-vocational teams." The pain is medically treated insofar as possible while the patient is retrained in work he can handle. Operant conditioning may be added to increase the level of activity.

How does the doctor distinguish between the outright fraud and the patient with real problems of pain behavior? One way, says Dr. Sternbach, is to impose a time limit on the dialogue. Very few pain patients are totally disabled. They are able to perform some kind of activity in spite of the pain. The patient who talks about returning to work can be pushed into agreeing to find something else to do if he is unable to handle his regular job, so a time limit is imposed upon him.

A different game is played by the drug-dependent patient who designs his play to ensure a regular supply of his analgesic medicines. Except for frank drug addicts, the usual pain patient does not admit to a dependency. In fact, he usually professes an aversion to taking medication and the game consists of exploring alternatives with the doctor along the lines of the "Yes, but—" game, in which every suggestion is regretfully found wanting, so that in the end they are forced to fall back again on the detested medication. Dr. Sternbach describes a fanciful dialogue:

"Doctor, when the pain came on last night I took some Talwin you gave me and it didn't work, so I took some codeine my friend had, and some Darvon that Dr. Pushover prescribed for me, and it eased the pain only a little bit. I hate taking all those pills. Can't you cut a nerve or something?"

The doctor recoils at the suggestion, argues it is not necessary at this stage, and is led into prescribing something a little stronger than the Talwin. If the new drug works better and provides something in the way of euphoria, the patient is soothed for the time, but the game is far from over. The supply line must be strengthened and maintained.

At the next interview he protests again about the pain and how hard it is to bear with it. The doctor asks if it is worse. No, it is better with the new drug, but taking medication all the time is awful, couldn't they operate instead? The doctor again backs away from surgery, feels he must offer something in its place, and says they had better keep on as they are going, so long as the new drug seems to be working. Which is exactly what the patient intended.

"When the patient protests so much," says Dr. Sternbach, "it is a good sign that an addiction problem is, in fact, brewing."

The way to stop it is to take the bull by the horns. On the next transaction, with the patient beginning again the familiar protest about hating to take all those pills and how he still hurts, the doctor abruptly agrees.

"You're right. The pills aren't doing that much good, and they can do you harm. Stop taking them."

This is not playing the game. The patient is thrown for a loss. "What do I do instead? What about the pain?"

"You're going to have to learn to live with it. If you can't stand it, take a couple of aspirins every four hours—no more."

That game is over. Unfortunately for the player he is dependent upon the doctor for his supply.

A third type is the patient Dr. Sternbach calls the Confounder. He is not interested in financial compensation nor in drugs, but in the sense of power that comes with proving the doctor wrong. The more celebrated the doctor is, the higher is the game payoff.

These patients are cooperative, follow instructions, show good initial response—and then the pain comes back. No matter what is done—surgery, medication, psychotherapy, or physical therapy, the pain always comes back.

The rules of the game call for complete responsiveness, which seduces the doctor into full involvement. Once he is completely committed, the patient lowers the boom. Failure.

The doctor might have felt a warning tingle as he read over the patient's medical history, with its record of earlier failures. But the patient is skillful.

"No one has been able to help me, doctor, but I am confident you will. Yours is the best program I've seen, and I've seen a lot of them. I feel sure you'll be able to help me."

The doctor is flattered in spite of himself. Besides, if conservative measures fail, he can always do a cordotomy. They fail, and he does. Success! The patient announces himself gloriously free of pain for the first time in years.

The congratulations are short-lived. In a few months the pain is back worse than ever. "Doctor, this is terrible. Can't you do something?"

Sometimes he can be pulled in for a second round. But if he is astute enough to become very suspicious at this point, salvation lies in a complete reversal of tactics. He offers no assurances.

"I don't know if I can help you. Probably not. In fact, looking over your medical history, I'd say we can't. It's going to be up to you from now on."

"Whatever you say, doctor." The patient doesn't take the threat very seriously. Give the doctor a little rope and he'll come in for another game.

So now the patient reports improvement. The gun-shy practitioner doesn't take the bait. "Let's see how long this lasts. I'm not at all confident that the pain won't come back. It always has. Let's wait and see."

The games, Dr. Sternbach says, illustrate a revelation that some chronic pain patients can and will manipulate and control their doctors out of a compulsion to remain as pain patients. The primary function of the pain game is to perpetuate that life-style and identity.

The doctor's defense against games is to refuse to play, but this is only part of the problem—the part of self-protection. To help the patient, he must now be prepared to offer realistic and acceptable alternatives to game playing.

What is difficult to grasp is the ambivalence of the long-time pain patient. On one level he is engaged in a game of painmanship, the object of which is to evade a cure, to produce in Dr. Sternbach's words, "undiagnosable pain and unrelievable suffering." It is apparently more satisfying to him to confound the doctor than to overcome the pain. This process, which challenges the doctor's identity as a healer, at the same time reinforces the patient's image of himself as *homo dolorosus.*

In his portrait of "the low-back loser," [4] Dr. Sternbach emphasizes the depression which lies beneath the surface of the patient with a history of back pain. It is usually concealed. The patient does not show signs of depression and may deny being depressed except by the pain. Yet his MMPI consistently shows above-normal depression. In their answers to questions on the Cornell Medical Index, low-back pain patients respond much more frequently than do arthritics to questions asking if they consider themselves sickly, or frequently ill, with a yes answer. They also indulge in twice as many pain games as patients with rheumatoid arthritis.

Still, there is a dichotomy here. The patient is really suffering, and is really asking for help. The doctor's problem is to find an approach that is acceptable. If he can find such an approach, even the long-time losers will at last give up their gamesmanship and their pain careers.

These patients are difficult to treat because a majority of this type are somatic, they translate depression or other neurotic problems into bodily symptoms including pain. The somatic patient is also a poor candidate for psychotherapy, clinging to the belief that there is something wrong with him that the doctor

[4] Richard A. Sternbach et al., "Chronic Low-Back Pain," *Postgraduate Medicine,* Vol. 53, No. 6, May 1973, pp. 135-38.

simply has not been able to discover. He is unconvinced by any suggestion that his pain has an emotional basis.

If the pain is of long duration, enough operant conditioning has occurred to make semi or total invalidism a fixed way of life, strongly resistant to change. Like the alcoholic, drug addict, or obese person, "these several kinds of chronic patients," says Dr. Sternbach, "who are in reality personality disorders, have all in effect 'opted out' or checked out of the social system with its involved relationships and commitments, and pain patients, like the others, strongly resist the coercion to get back in."[5]

One approach to cracking this Berlin Wall has been called contract psychiatry, or as Dr. Sternbach calls it, the "treatment contract."

The doctor adopts a no-nonsense, blunt approach. He is aware that this type of patient is neither verbal nor imaginative and is therefore not impressed by theory or psychological suggestion. He thinks in action terms. The doctor cuts through his defenses by offering him a treatment contract couched in specific action terms.

He begins by asking the patient if he really wants to be cured of his pain, and if he is willing to work at it. If the answer is "no," the whole business would end right there, the doctor would go no further.

But this is rare; the great majority say, "Yes, of course." The doctor does not take the statement at face value. It is too easy to say yes. He points out, bluntly and tactlessly, that pain now occupies a large role in the patient's life-style and that to give it up will take courage in starting treatment that could be unpleasant and certainly will be hard work.

"We add quickly that we will not, and could not if we wanted to, take his pain away from him, but we can help him give up his pain if that is what he decides to do."

This kind of bluntness, says Dr. Sternbach, is not often well received. The patient becomes pathetic and stubborn, goes into a recital of his pain symptoms and a history of his medical findings, brings up the contradictions in the things he has been told, with the obvious implication that doctors are either inept or untrustworthy, and shows resentment at the implication that he can

[5] Richard A. Sternbach and Thomas N. Rusk, "Alternatives to the Pain Career," *Psychotherapy: Theory, Research, and Practice,* forthcoming.

"give up" his pain, as though it were something created out of his imagination.

The doctor cuts him off, saying he is not interested in this past history and will not discuss it. He repeats his question: "Do you want to get rid of your pain and will you work with us, in our way, to do so?"

Resistance may have to be beaten down, and there may be several repetitions of this before the patient may finally agree. Then the contract is laid out in explicit detail.

It is explained that if the patient decides to give up his pain, his life will change radically, and this may not be as easy as one might think. "How do you propose to live when the pain is gone? You've spent years adapting your life to it, how will you fill its place? What will you do? What ambitions or goals will you set for yourself? Will that be enough for you? Will it meet all your needs?"

Even blunter is the dissection of the pain rewards the patient has been cultivating. The doctor forces a hard look at the pay-offs in the pain career, what the patient will be giving up if he changes, and what alternatives there are to replace these dubious satisfactions.

The patient must agree to begin new activities outside his hospital therapy, such as looking for some kind of work or equivalent activity, and to report back on his progress.

Finally he is told he will be put on antidepressant medication rather than the narcotic/analgesic, or whatever he had been taking.

In return, the doctor unfolds his part of the contract. He will guarantee improvement if the patient achieves the goals of the contract. He also guarantees the pain will worsen if the patient rejects the contract or cheats on the terms.

This is no idle threat, Dr. Sternbach says. "In our experience the pain diminishes in rough proportion to the success with which the patient behaves in accordance with his alternative pain-free life-style, and even if there is an organic pain generator which is not surgically correctable, the pain level decreases to a point which the patient can live with."

But experience has also shown that if the patient does cheat, he is likely to resort to operation after operation which bring no relief, to drugs which are addictive, and to run the great risk of winding up bedridden, crippled, addicted, but still in pain.

The contract lays out three specifics: the new goals of behavior the patient must adopt to be free of pain, the steps which need to be taken to reach these goals in spite of his pain, and the need to break through the patient's inertia or outright resistance to change.

There is still a good deal of testing, since the doctor knows that glib answers are also a way of life for professional pain patients. So probing questions continue to be asked.

"If you were free of pain, how would you live? What would you do?"

"I'd go back to work."

"Why would you do that? Was your job that interesting?"

"No, but it beats sitting around and hurting. Besides, did you ever try to live on my disability payments, doc?"

The protests of wanting to go back to work are automatic. The patient has absorbed enough hints that he is goldbricking that he feels a need to protest that his intentions are pure. The doctor doesn't let up on him.

"I don't think working in a fish market sounds like fun. And the salary can't be much better than welfare. Wouldn't you honestly be better off taking it easy and collecting your disability checks? You can get by without working. Are you sure you're not saying you want to work just because your family expects you to work? Be honest now, if it weren't for them, would you want to work?"

The patient may have no idea that a job is involved with his sense of identity, but he knows that being self-supporting brings more respect than being supported. The doctor's purpose is to challenge his assertions, to shake them if they are flimsy, make him support them or change them until they are shaken down to those about which he can show interest and enthusiasm. They must be goals which are attainable, not a glib recitation of wholly insincere aims that he parrots because he knows what is expected.

Dr. Sternbach says that to his surprise he often has to push hard on the notion of human relationships, that many or most of the patients seem not to want to talk about family or friends, and do not seem greatly interested in making or keeping relationships. Many are loners, unmarried, divorced, widowed, or in flight from an unhappy relationship. They do not seem to have close friends.

The doctor points out that pain has become a constant companion, familiar if not joyful, and to give it up demands a substitute—something or someone to fill the hours hitherto devoted to it. It may actually be easier to live with the pain than to face the prospect of rejection if one of the goals is the making of new relationships.

Out of this testing and retesting of stated goals may evolve a few that the patient will stick with and work to attain. Typical might be goals in three areas: work, human contacts, and recreation. Thus he may agree to complete a certain amount of work on a rehabilitation program or, if able to get about, to find some outside work; to see some friend every day; and to do something in the way of recreation—walk, fish, play golf, or whatever.

Progress is not expected to be rapid. If it is broken down into recognizable steps, progress can be measured. These steps might be called subcontracts. For a really withdrawn patient the act of making a phone call or writing a letter or inquiring about a study class is an achievement, and brings him a step closer to the kind of activity he needs.

This is what Dr. Fordyce would call well-behavior as contrasted with sick-behavior. Such behavior is inconsistent with the pain state and expands the time spent in a state of no-pain. If the patient balks at beginning this kind of behavior it is an indication that he is still not committed to the contract, and his resistance may force termination.

The well-behavior is also reinforced by reviewing the patient's activities, going over what he has done since the previous session, and encouraging him in the correct kind of behavior.

In discussions between doctor and patient the doctor avoids generalities, tries to be as explicit as possible, and concentrates on specific behavioral goals. This makes it possible to chart progress step by step and to substitute recognizable activity for rhetoric. It makes it possible to deal with covert resistance by pointing out that although the patient has insisted upon his desire to increase certain activities, like seeing friends, he has actually found one reason after another for avoiding it.

Identifying such resistance, the doctor suggests they end the therapy since the patient is obviously not fulfilling his part of the contract. Being thus attacked, the patient will normally defend himself by protesting that he has every intention of going through with the contract, it is just that circumstances have conspired against him.

The doctor replies that a cardinal rule of all relationships is to pay less attention to what people say than to what they do, and the patient simply hasn't done it. He is not only trying to fool the doctor, he is fooling himself, which he is welcome to do but not on the doctor's time.

This kind of tough treatment is apparently necessary, for resistance commonly appears after the first few months of therapy. It occurs in a learning plateau when the patient has achieved some insight but has not yet reached the point of translating it into behavior change. It needs to be dealt with immediately.

In fact, says Dr. Sternbach, it is better for the patient to develop new behavior habits without insight than to have insight and not act upon it.

Resistance is also shown in talk sessions with the therapist, when the patient indulges in a voluptuous orgy of describing his pains, symptoms, operations, and all the gossip surrounding his condition and its treatment. This is common in hypochondria where the patient shows all too clearly that his major interest in life is his disability and his pain. The only real enthusiasm he ever displays is in discussing the very thing he insists he wants to be rid of permanently.

The doctor brings him up short by pointing out the waste in channeling all his talents into complaints, that this is giving him an unhealthy satisfaction and how obviously difficult it is for him to give it up. The doctor himself intends to forego this luxury of recall because frankly it has become a crashing bore, because it is imperative for the patient to forget this kind of satisfaction and look for healthier outlets, and finally because these monologues do nothing but delay the actual therapy, which is working toward the goals of the contract. From here on, sympathy is out and the doctor will refuse to tolerate any indulgence in self-pity.

There is, in fact, a real-life struggle between patient and doctor. The patient resists change, clings to his pain, while he does in fact wish to be free of it. His ambivalence is built around the fear of change and the lack of something constructive to replace the pain career. The doctor offers him a better life-style and a means of gaining it: the contract, which specifies explicitly the goals. Success, says Dr. Sternbach, depends upon the patient's complete cooperation in carrying out the step-by-step methods laid out and in giving up his resistance.

An extremely effective technique in overcoming resistance and game-playing is exposure by other patients. "Many games and payoffs are not consciously conceived of by patients, and their exposure by other patients who have participated in the same type of game-playing is frequently more effective than when done by the staff." [6]

A doctor hesitates to say to a patient, "Come on now, you're not hurting as much as you protest—you can get off your butt and walk if you want to!"

The patient has considerable justification in snapping back, "That's pretty easy for you to say, doc. You're not hurting!"

But if another patient in obviously worse condition says the same thing, it hits home. Patients may fool the staff, says Dr. Sternbach, but they don't fool other patients very long. Exposing the game and its payoffs to the wife of the patient who has been the victim of these games for years is an eye-opener for her. If she decides to stop playing, it is a great advantage in checking the old games and aborting the formation of new games.

[6] Jerry H. Greenhoot and Richard A. Sternbach, "Conjoint Treatment of Chronic Pain," *International Symposium on Pain*.

Chapter 12

THE HEADACHE CLINIC

The whole patient, not the symptom, is the single
most important factor in the treatment of headache.
ARNOLD P. FRIEDMAN, M.D. *

Headache is so common that physicians estimate it to be the major complaint in more than half the number of patients who come to their offices. Yet one specialist, Dr. Raymond L. Hilsinger,** who believes that 140 million Americans suffer from one or more forms of headache at varying times, also thinks that not more than 10 percent of them go to see their doctors about it.

As in all pain problems, an infrequent headache is one thing, a chronic, recurring headache is something else. Ruling out any serious underlying pathology, it is still possible to have headaches of such blinding pain that life becomes a torment.

There is nothing enviable about such a situation, but if you have headaches, it may be a small consolation to know that you are in good company. Some of the most brilliant and celebrated

---

* "Treatment of Headache," *International Journal of Neurology*, Vol. 9, No. 1, 1972, pp. 11-22. Dr. Friedman is now retired. He was formerly Physician in Charge, Headache Unit, Division of Neurology, Montefiore Hospital, New York.
** Associate Clinical Professor, Department of Otolaryngology, College of Medicine, University of Cincinnati, Cincinnati, Ohio.

people of history were tormented by migraine to such an extent
that their creative productivity is a source of wonder.

The worst victim may have been Friedrich Nietzsche, philosopher of sorts and intellectual parent of Superman. Nietzsche's
headaches were so frequent that in their peak period they were
coming about every seventy-two hours, with 118 attacks in a
single year. Evidently there was some underlying pathology because ill health forced him to resign his professorship at Basel
when he was only thirty-five, and he became insane ten years
later.

Charles Darwin was another migraine sufferer. He was a loner,
a sensitive, turned-in man. As a boy, he was so cowed by a tyran-
nical father that he acquired a permanent expression of apology
for not ever measuring up to his father's expectations, a situation which undoubtedly created in him a chronic feeling of guilt
that he carried all his life. He was convinced that his migraine
was genetic, for he referred to it as a "hereditary" illness and, in
fact, it did seem to be passed on to three of his children.

Sigmund Freud had headaches, which he himself diagnosed
as migraine and, since he was a neurologist, he was in a position
to know. About 1899 he had frequent attacks, but a year later
wrote to a colleague that he was better, with only a "slight migraine on Sundays."

The record shows two American presidents who had firsthand
experience with migraine: Thomas Jefferson and Ulysses S.
Grant. Jefferson has mentioned in his journals that his headaches
were not frequent—probably at intervals of several years—but
when they did happen they were severe. A letter dated 1790
refers to a headache which lasted a week and left him "unable as
yet to write or read without great pain."

Another reference in 1808 speaks of a headache in its tenth
day. Yet he referred to the pain as "very moderate and yesterday
did not last more than three hours."

As is often the case with migraine, the attacks became milder
as Jefferson got older and apparently ended altogether at last.
In 1819, when he was seventy-six years old, he wrote to a friend
that the headaches which had plagued him every six or eight
years for two or three weeks at a time now seemed to have left
him for good.

Grant was neither the philosopher nor writer that Jefferson was, but he did keep a journal and in it he recorded a sick headache that unhorsed him on the eve of Lee's surrender. The pain was so intense that he stopped at a farmhouse behind the main body of his troops to rest.

"I spent the night in bathing my feet in hot water and mustard, and putting mustard plasters on my wrists and the back part of my neck, hoping to be cured by morning." Morning came but the headache was not gone. Then a messenger brought a note from Lee. He had the day before refused to surrender but now was ready to accept Grant's terms. The news cured Grant's headache immediately. "The pain in my head seemed to leave me the moment I got Lee's letter."

Dr. Arnold P. Friedman, whose career has included operating the headache unit at Montefiore Hospital in New York, and being Clinical Professor of Neurology at Columbia University, has collected a list of some famous migraine sufferers. He includes, in addition to those already mentioned, John Calvin, Madame Pompadour, Karl Marx, the Duke of Marlborough, Alfred Nobel, and Mary Todd Lincoln.

Going further back in time, headaches were familiar to the ancient Mesopotamians around 4000 B.C. and the Sumerians about 8000 B.C. The Greeks and Romans knew migraine well. The Greeks considered the pain to be caused by Keres—evil spirits—which Aristotle believed entered a man's stomach and sent "humours" up to the brain, with the well-known results.

The Romans modernized this evil spirit theory, speculating that he who acquired a headache had offended a touchy god and was being punished for it. The word "pain," in fact, comes from the Latin *poena* which means, literally, punishment.

The famous Roman physician Galen apparently was influenced by Greek science, for he held that headaches were caused by the "ascent of vapors" which would be too hot or too cold, or just too much.

The devil theory led to the usual remedies, each highly touted by its own advocates—a tuft of hair from a virgin kid, a snakeskin, moss scraped from a statue, a common weed called plantain, a decapitated bird, garlic, a hot iron, dill, snuff, or just putting a hangman's noose around the neck. This last, if tightened, was a sure cure for headache. And, of course, there was prayer, magic, and charms replete with such ingredients as live toads, lizards, and bats.

Herbal remedies persisted down to modern times; in fact, they are still popular in many parts of the world. Mugwort and wormwood were well thought of, as was a solution of wild geranium to be applied to the head. Flowers were popular. A seventeenth-century list of headache remedies from France includes the rose, geranium, and poppy, as well as marjoram and walnuts.

Tobacco in the form of snuff was thought to be a specific cure for headache. *Cantharides* or Spanish fly, powdered and dried, and mixed with vinegar and "leaven," was placed on the skin and allowed to raise blisters, the theory being that when the blister was opened and the clear liquid drained out, the pain would drain out with it.

With this very brief look at the unwholesome history of headache, let us define our terms. Every pain in the head is not a headache.

"To the patient, headache is a disease, but to the physician it is only a symptom, a symptom of an illness which may be either organic or functional. In the vast majority of cases it will prove to be of functional origin." [1]

A functional illness is one that affects the function but not the structure of the organ involved. The layman may be relieved to know that his tissues are not being eroded, but to the physician it is still an illness.

Pain in the head may emanate from tissues outside or inside the skull. Outside the skull are skin, scalp, muscles, mucous membranes, fascia (the bands of fibrous tissue that enclose muscles and organs), arteries, and veins. All are sensitive to pain, especially the arteries.

Inside the cranium are sinuses, arteries, veins, and parts of the dura mater, the outer tough membrane that covers brain and spinal cord. In addition there are the nerves of the head, the trigeminal, facial, glossopharyngeal, vagal, second and third cervical nerves. These, of course, are directly involved with pain.

Head pains may be superficial, such as those resulting from irritation of the skin or mucous membranes. They may be neural-

[1] B. T. Horton, "Management of Vascular Headaches," *Angiology*, Vol. 10, No. 1, February 1959, pp. 43-56.

gic, affecting the nerves mentioned, in which case the pain is usually described as "burning" or "tearing," but of short duration. And finally there is cephalgia, or headache, which is deep, usually dull rather than sharp, not localized as other types of pain, and prolonged over hours or days. The true headache results from a stimulation of cranial muscles or blood vessels, or some of the sensitive organs inside the skull.

Any persistent head pain should, of course, be checked out. The physician takes a headache history, asking questions to familiarize himself with the pattern of onset, frequency, location, degree of severity, warning symptoms, other symptoms that might occur in association with the headache, and how it has affected the patient's behavior and sleep. This should be followed by a physical and neurological examination and skull film to rule out the unlikely chance of brain tumor. Only where there is a suspicion of organic disease does the physician go on to brain scan, spinal tap, angiogram, pneumoencephalogram, and so on.

There are various ways of classifying headaches; one prepared by the Committee on Classification of Headache of the National Institute of Neurological Diseases and Blindness, of which Dr. Friedman has been chairman, is as follows:

1. **Migraine**
   Migraine variants
   Vascular headache
   Atypical facial neuralgia

2. **Tension headache**

3. **Intercranial disturbances**
   Arteriosclerosis
   Vascular anomalies
   Aneurysms
   Tumor
   Infections

4. **Extracranial disturbances**
   Eye
   Ear
   Nose
   Bones of skull and neck

5. **Cranial trauma**

6. Systemic disease
   Hypertension
   Allergy
   Arteritis
   Fever
   Infection

7. Psychogenic headache
   Conversion
   Tension

Dr. Seymour Diamond* uses a somewhat different method of classification, modified from that of the American Association for the Study of Headache and the World Federation of Neurology's Research Group on Migraine and Headache. He lists three major classes of headache: vascular, muscle contraction, and traction and inflammatory.

Vascular headaches include migraines, cluster, hypertensive, and a few others, in all comprising 50 percent of those seen. The muscle contraction or tension class, which includes anxiety and depression headaches, amounts to 48 percent, and those caused by a number of disease conditions under the traction and inflammatory heading are no more than 2 percent.

There has been a change in the pattern of headache seen at the clinic in Chicago's Mt. Sinai Hospital, says Dr. Diamond. "When we first opened the clinic, 75 to 85 percent of the patients had headaches of psychogenic origin. Headache as a symptom of depression has not been well recognized and the relief is more difficult because the patient doesn't respond to the usual analgesics. Our recent analysis of more than 1,000 patients with headache (seen over the past two years) shows a shift in statistics so that vascular headaches and headaches of psychogenic origin both have an occurrence rate of about 50 percent." [2]

* Clinical Assistant Professor in Neurology, Chicago Medical School; Chairman, Department of Family Medicine, St. Joseph Hospital; Co-Director, Headache Clinic, Mt. Sinai Hospital Medical Center, Chicago, Illinois; President, National Migraine Foundation; Executive Secretary, American Association for the Study of Headache.

[2] Seymour Diamond and Bernard J. Baltes, "Management of Headache by the Family Physician," *American Family Physician*, Vol. 5, No. 4, April 1972, pp. 68-76. Bernard J. Baltes, M.D., Ph.D., is Co-Director of the Headache Clinic at Mt. Sinai, Chairman of Pharmacy and Research Committee at St. Joseph Hospital; Vice-President Clinical Research, Samuel H. Flamm Research Foundation, Chicago, Illinois.

Dr. Friedman says, "In 85 to 90 percent of cases of chronic recurrent headaches, the attack is vascular headache of the migraine type or of the muscle contraction (tension) type, or a combination of these."

What is a vascular headache? The term "vascular" applies, of course, to the blood vessels. Apparently an attack is preceded by a constriction of the intercranial arteries. Then, as the headache begins, the arteries dilate and there is an inflammation of the arterial wall from the accumulation of two chemical substances—bradykinin and serotonin.

While no one seems to know exactly what causes the headache, there is a general feeling that it is associated with a following sudden drop of serotonin in the blood. One reason to think so is that the drug reserpine, which depletes serotonin in the blood platelets, can bring on a migraine headache in susceptible people —but not in normal people. And an injection of serotonin can relieve migraine attacks whether they are spontaneous or induced.

There are premonitory symptoms, called prodromes. One prodrome is an "aura," an eerie, psychic sensation of something about to happen. Another involves visual disturbances—flashes of light or intolerance to light. A blind spot may appear; looking at a page of type, the patient may see only half of it, or a jagged round hole may open in the page in which the type disappears. These symptoms occur during the vasoconstrictive phase.

With the second phase, vasodilation, one side of the head begins to throb and the pain builds sharply to an excruciating peak. At the height of the attack there is a good deal of nausea and vomiting and extreme irritability. Although lying down brings slight relief, the pain may last for days.

In the third phase the blood vessels become swollen and distended, with a pipelike rigidity. The pain becomes dull and steady rather than throbbing. Muscle tension in the head and neck may now add its own type of pain and this may persist beyond the original headache.

Common migraine produces symptoms generally like those already described. The pain usually starts in the morning, as the patient awakes, although he may be awakened by the headache. The pain builds over the next several hours and is usually unilateral (on one side of the head). Frequently the eye on that side tears, and the nasal passage on the same side becomes congested. Nausea, vomiting, diarrhea, and chills follow. The attack may last for days.

Classic migraine is slightly different. Where the prodromes in common migraine are vague, they are sharply defined in classic migraine, usually visual, although motor control can be affected too. But blind spots are the most frequent symptom, and they usually occur on the side opposite to the head pain. The pain is unilateral but tends to alternate sides in different attacks. The pain builds in an hour and generally lasts for four to six hours rather than days as in common migraine. Nausea and vomiting frequently occur, although not invariably.

Cluster headache (histaminic cephalgia, or Horton's syndrome) is a series of migraine attacks coming in groups or clusters, usually close together and usually at the same time each day. The attack begins with a burning sensation in one eye or in the temple. The eye tears copiously and the burning discomfort, which lasts only a few minutes, is followed by intense pain, either throbbing or steady. There is nasal stuffiness on the same side. The pain may last for as little as fifteen minutes or as long as four hours, but generally not longer than this. The cluster headache is the most intense pain of all headaches. It usually begins at night, waking the patient out of sleep. This is a different pattern from ordinary migraine or the common emotional headache, in which the patient awakens with a sense of discomfort and presently realizes his head hurts. In cluster headache the pain is so agonizing that it shocks the patient out of sleep. He cannot lie still but is driven to his feet in reaction to the pain. He must get up and do something, says Dr. Diamond, "walk, cry, scream, or even beat his head."

A characteristic of cluster migraine is that there may be remissions in which the headaches totally disappear for months or even years, but eventually return.

There are in all some five variations of the migraine headache, the others less common, but all unpleasant. Since all are vascular headaches, treatment is aimed at constricting the dilated blood vessels.

What kind of individual is subject to migraine? For one thing, it may begin at any age. In some 25 percent of patients it begins as early as age ten. People over 45 rarely experience migraine for the first time, although if it is present, it can continue into the fifties. About 65 percent of migraine sufferers have a family history of headache and more women are affected than men.

The medical histories of many patients combine to show a psychological profile of a rigid individual, a perfectionist, often with a family background noted for stiff-upper-lip pride and inflexible standards of behavior. The members of the family tend to be reserved and undemonstrative, unforgiving when they consider themselves wronged. Any deviation from the family standard is coldly punished. Rebels are forced to suppress their defiance or face ostracism, so usually go underground and accumulate feelings of hostility and guilt. There seems to be a correlation between the pressure directed at them and the headaches.

The typical migraine patient, then, is the rigid, compulsive perfectionist whose own emotions, moods, and fears are guiltily suppressed. Such a psychological profile obviously can lead to a variety of neuroses; in some individuals it is expressed in headaches.

Tension headache, or muscle contraction headache, is linked to periods of stress. A family history of headache is not so much a factor as with migraine. The headaches fluctuate with the stress periods of the individual, and usually one of the attacks occurs when the stress is at its peak, or just afterward. These headaches are more common in women than in men, and they may be the type of headache most frequently encountered in a doctor's practice.

An analysis of 1,000 cases by Dr. Friedman indicated that the largest number of patients reported these headaches between the ages of twenty and forty years. Thirty percent said their headaches were a daily occurrence and 20 percent claimed constant headache.

The pain is usually bilateral—on both sides of the head. It is sometimes described as actual pain, sometimes as merely pressure, a feeling like a tight band around the head. It may go on all day with the patient never free of discomfort except with drugs. He may get to sleep but awake in the morning with the headache still there, and this pattern may continue for months or even years. The pain is dull but constant and debilitating, and a complete irritant. If anything good can be said about it, perhaps it is only that there is an absence of the nausea and vomiting that accompanies migraine.

Frequently there is spasm of the skeletal muscles which leads to a complaint of "sore neck." Or the patient may clench his teeth and complain of aching jaw muscles.

There are a number of disease conditions which can produce muscle contraction headache—infection or inflammation of the muscles, bony abnormalities and disorders of the temporomandibular joint—the hinge of the lower jaw. Chewing aggravates this pain and it usually requires correction of the bite by a dentist with, sometimes, the additional relief obtained by nerve block.

The depressive headache is fairly common. Dr. Diamond says that about 48 percent of the patients coming to the clinic have a psychogenic basis for their pain. The majority of these, as many as 85 percent, are experiencing a conversion reaction, with their emotional conflicts—hostility or self-dislike—converted into pain.

A telltale symptom in depressive headache is the patient's feeling that he has had these headaches all his life, or at least for many years. His sleep is disturbed; he tends to waken during the night and to be up early, with the headache feeling worse in the morning. Another clue is that the depressive headache does not respond to the usual analgesic drugs.

Headache can also result from pathological causes: high blood pressure, glaucoma, or angioma—a tumor made up of blood or lymph vessels, for which reason persistent headache should always be checked out.

But for headache pure and simple, the conservative treatment consists of drugs and psychotherapy. Headache is always a symptom, and treatment needs to be directed at the whole patient rather than just the symptom. Once he is through the medical and neurological examinations, the doctor considers the personality of the patient and the environment in which he lives and works. To a perceptive diagnostician, the cause may be clearly apparent in the patient's life-style and the stresses surrounding him.

Of course the doctor has little control over his patient's life-style, and he can only make suggestions or threaten consequences if the factors he recognizes as damaging are not changed or removed.

Some changes he can make. For example, in some people a migraine attack can be caused by an amino acid, tyramine, which is present in chocolate, some cheeses, citrus fruits, fried foods, onions, tea, coffee, pork, seafood, and alcohol. Another chemical discovered to trigger headache is monosodium glutamate, a flavor enhancer much in favor in the Chinese school of cookery, so much so that "Chinese restaurant syndrome" became a byword not long ago. Susceptible people complained of head and neck pains after eating a meal in a Chinese restaurant. Migraine sufferers have learned to avoid these foods, as well as alcohol and cigarettes.

The doctor can help here by making practical suggestions about regulation of mealtimes and being careful to avoid other predisposing factors such as too bright or flickering lights, motion sickness, and so on.

Antidepressants of the MAO (monoamine oxidase inhibitor) type are also known to trigger migraine, especially in combination with a tyramine-containing food which sends the blood pressure sky-high and creates frightening headache even in people not subject to migraine.

Hormones such as estrogen and progesterone can also set off a migraine attack, and women susceptible to migraine need to consider this in relation to the birth control pill. "In some patients," says Dr. J. D. Carroll,* "undoubtedly the contraceptive pill produces a deterioration in their migraine, taking the form of either an increase in the frequency or severity of the attacks, or both." [3]

He also notes that migraine clears up completely in pregnancy for about 80 percent of patients but returns a few weeks after delivery.

As to psychotherapy, the average physician, unless he happens to have psychiatric training, is limited to supportive counseling, offering encouragement, advice, and a listening ear. The

* M.D., F.R.C.P. Ed., Consulting Neurologist, Royal County Hospital, Guildford, Surrey, England.
[3] "Migraine—General Management," *British Medical Journal,* Vol. 2, 1971, pp. 756-7.

advice generally is aimed at the patient's low opinion of himself and his fruitless quest for perfection, reminding him how impossible this goal is, and that his compulsiveness is destructive.

The migraine patient needs support in refusing to accept an overload of responsibility, to be reminded that he cannot please everyone and that realistically he should stop trying so hard. He also needs to stop feeling guilty, to stop deprecating himself, and to start liking himself a little better.

Drug treatment for migraine is on two levels—aborting the attack if it has begun, and prophylaxis between attacks to reduce the frequency and severity of the headaches when they do come.

For aborting a migraine headache, the drug of choice is ergotamine tartrate, available under brand names such as Cafergot or Ergomar. The first includes caffeine, which increases the constrictive effect on the blood vessels and, in Dr. Friedman's opinion, reduces the amount of ergotamine required. One or two milligrams is given at the start, then two milligrams every hour, with six milligrams maximum in any attack and not more than ten a week.

An injectable form of ergotamine, D.H.E. 45, is used for very rapid action, and limited to three cubic centimeters a day. Gynergen is another injectable form for stopping the acute attack; its use is limited to two cubic centimeters a week.

These warnings on dosage are real. Ergotamine can be addictive if patients use it daily and, with developing tolerance, increase the dosage over a period of time.

Prophylactic treatment calls for a different drug or variety of drugs. The most effective is considered to be methysergide maleate, brand name Sansert, with a success rating of 55 to 65 percent. Sansert works by deactivating serotonin and histamine. It has some possible unpleasant side effects including muscle cramps and abdominal discomfort, but more serious, has been known to produce fibrotic changes in the heart. It is therefore used no longer than six months at a stretch without a rest period of six to eight weeks for any possible toxicity to disperse.

Other drugs used for prophylaxis are numerous; they include phenobarbital, tranquilizers, antihistamines, antidepressants, and the anticonvulsant Dilantin. This group, according to Dr. Friedman, has a success rate of 35 to 40 percent—about the same as a placebo.

The Headache Clinic 135

The role of the autonomic nervous system is stressed by Dr. Hilsinger. The autonomic system in every human being controls involuntary functions like breathing, heartbeat, digestion, the action of glands, and the circulation.

The autonomic system is divided into two parts: the sympathetic and the parasympathetic divisions. "They exist," says Dr. Hilsinger, "in a state of balanced opposition in order to maintain a stable internal bodily environment. There is reason to believe that autonomic imbalance may be implicated in the genesis of headache. Autonomic pathways are involved in the vasodilating process observed in headaches." [4]

Over the past eighteen years, Dr. Hilsinger has treated more than 5,000 headache patients with Bellergal, a compound containing ergotamine tartrate and belladonna. Another form, Bellergal Spacetabs, adds phenobarbital. The action of the ergotamine on the blood vessels is reinforced by the action of belladonna as an inhibitor of the sympathetic and parasympathetic systems, and of phenobarbital as a general dampening influence of the cortical centers.

Taken twice a day, this medication is believed by Dr. Hilsinger to lengthen the intervals between headaches and decrease the severity of the pain should an attack still take place.

Simple tranquilizers like Librium, Valium, Atarax, or Vistaril also have a dampening effect on undesirable nerve impulses, particularly for tension headaches.

To drugs and psychotherapy, Dr. Friedman would add physiotherapy for helping tightened muscles to relax. This would include massage, hot packs or immersion of neck and head in warm water, and even neck traction. Such measures, he says, are temporary but in some patients where there is a structural difficulty of the muscles, joints, or fibrous tissues, the proper treatment can produce long-lasting improvement.

For the depressed patient suffering from the depressive headache, a number of drugs are available—Elavil, Tofranil, Norpramin, Aventyl, and Vivactil. Ordinarily, tranquilizers are not used for the depressed patient as they tend to increase the depression. However there is often an underlying anxiety masked

[4] "Chronic Recurring Headache: Symptoms, Diagnosis, Treatment," a scientific exhibit at the American Medical Association Annual Convention, New York, June 23-27, 1973.

by the depression, and the anxiety-calming effect of a tranquilizer is desirable. In such a case the physician may combine a tranquilizer with an antidepressant, or use a new drug, Sinequan, which combines both actions in a single entity.

A slightly sour note on the drug scene comes from England. Discussing new research in migraine, Dr. J. N. Blau takes a slightly skeptical look at some of the medications in use.[5] *Any* therapeutic trial in migraine, he says, usually shows an improvement rate of about 60 percent, no matter *what* is used.

"It must be self-evident that ergotamine preparations are not the final answer. Many physicians I know take only aspirin or another analgesic for their own migraine. Even those patients helped by ergot find that only after the drug has made them vomit do they obtain relief, and it is well recognized that vomiting can end an attack. Often the drug remains unabsorbed in the stomach, owing to gastric stasis. Many proprietary preparations contain a sedative, analgesic, or a stimulant, in addition to ergot. All in all, the interpretation of the results of a therapeutic trial for migraine is fraught with difficulties."

Writing in the same issue, June 26, 1971, of the *British Medical Journal,* Dr. Marcia Wilkinson, Medical Director of the City Migraine Clinic of St. Bartholomew's Hospital in London, says, "Probably more patients with migraine are helped by simple analgesics than by any other type of therapy, and these should be tried before any other treatment is given." By simple analgesics she means of course the ubiquitous aspirin.

Even more critical in another paper was W. E. Waters, M.B., B.S., D.I.H., of the Scientific Staff, Medical Research Council's Epidemiology Unit (South Wales), Cardiff. Dr. Waters performed a double-blind controlled study of 88 women "identified during a community survey as having headaches with the features of migraine."[6]

Seventy-nine of the women completed the trials, and of these, 40 gained relief from oral administration of ergotamine tartrate and 46 benefited from a placebo. "There was no evidence that ergotamine in doses of two or three milligrams was more effective than the placebo. Ergotamine aggravated the attack significantly

[5] "Migraine Research," *British Medical Journal,* Vol. 2, 1971, pp. 751-4.
[6] "Controlled Clinical Trial of Ergotamine Tartrate," *British Medical Journal,* Vol. 2, 1970, pp. 325-7.

more often than the placebo. Neither the color of the tablets nor the order of therapy significantly affected the results of the treatment."

This is a curious finding, inasmuch as ergotamine is so much the drug of choice for migraine, so specific in action, that it is actually used to help diagnose the condition. In other words, if ergotamine brings relief, the headache must be migraine.

In accepting the orthodoxy of ergotamine as the drug of choice in treating migraine, there is a danger that Dr. Waters characterizes as "circular definition," whereby migraine is a headache due to vasodilation and ergotamine is highly specific because of its vasoconstrictor action. The fallacy, he says, is that ergotamine was originally used when migraine was believed to be due to a spasm of cranial arteries, and acted by producing arterial relaxation. Today it is given for the opposite reason.

One element stands out. All the authorities agree on the importance of the psychological factors in headache. In spite of all the physical conditions or incidents which may conspire to bring on a migraine attack, the emotional factor is the most common. And so, says Dr. Friedman, treatment of the patient's psychological problems is paramount.

Says Dr. J. D. Carroll, "Migraine is a multifactorial disorder and it is most important that each patient should be carefully analyzed in the first instance from many aspects. The importance of a good doctor-patient relationship cannot be stressed too often, for this is a condition where psychological rapport is of great value and could well influence the success of treatment. Fortunately, also, a good ultimate prognosis can usually be given, for in most patients, the attacks tend to disappear with advancing age." [7]

Considering then that even conservative physicians stress the psychological factor, it is not at all surprising that less orthodox methods are being actively tried. One is an old and sometimes controversial tactic—hypnotism. The second is new and is creating excitement in some circles—biofeedback. We shall have a look at each.

[7] "Migraine—General Management," *British Medical Journal*, Vol. 2, 1971, pp. 756-7.

Chapter 13

HYPNOSIS

A state of increased receptivity to suggestion and direction, initially induced by the influence of another person. Often characterized by an altered state of consciousness, similar to that observed in spontaneous dissociative conditions. The degree may vary from mild hypersuggestibility to a trance state with complete surgical anesthesia.

A Psychiatric Glossary—
AMERICAN PSYCHIATRIC ASSOCIATION

That hypnosis is capable of producing complete anesthesia has been amply demonstrated. Major surgery, such as the removal of a lung, has been performed with no other anesthetic than hypnosis. The patient in one such lung operation, who was wide awake throughout, thought the surgeon was drawing a pencil line on his chest and wondered a little at it. What he had actually felt was the scalpel cutting through his chest wall.

Throughout this book the theme has recurred that pain is not a simple perceptual event, it is an emotional experience. Hypnosis is aimed directly at this emotional center. Explanations of how hypnosis changes emotion are not as simple as those which account for the effect of opiates, but there are some.

Speaking at the Seattle pain symposium, Dr. Martin T. Orne* suggested at least two different mechanisms.[1]

* M.D., Ph.D., Professor of Psychiatry, Director of Unit for Experimental Psychiatry, Institute of the Pennsylvania Hospital and University of Pennsylvania, Philadelphia.
[1] "Pain Suppression by Hypnosis and Related Phenomena," in press.

One, he said, was related to the placebo response. In essence, the patient expects something to happen, ergo, it tends to happen. This is obviously suggestion, but Dr. Orne noted that the effect was essentially not related to the extent of the hypnotic response, which one might interpret to mean that the patient is willing or eager to carry on and amplify even a slight influence exerted by the hypnotist.

The second mechanism suggested was a distortion of pain perception, on the order of negative hallucination. The two theories do not exclude each other. They can, in fact, be operating at the same time, independent but reinforcing each other.

Hypnotic analgesia, said Dr. Orne, does not seem to prevent the subject from having some reflex response to a painful stimulus. Stick a pin in him and you may get a muscle response. The real change there is that hypnosis has altered one of the reactive components connected with pain—anxiety.

This should sound familiar. You have heard the action of morphine described this way—that it affects the anxiety rather than the pain. In the case of hypnosis, said Dr. Orne, while many patients claimed they felt no pain, a number of objective tests indicated that they indeed did perceive pain, but were obviously quite able to ignore it.

At the same symposium in Seattle, Dr. Basil Finer[*] reiterated that the effect of hypnosis is to produce partial or complete detachment from anxiety, stress, and pain.[2]

Hypnosis is useful, he said, for the management of both acute and chronic pain. Some neurologists consider it helpful for the short term, but not for long-lasting chronic pain. But in Dr. Finer's experience, hypnosis has been used prophylactically as a preparation for future pain, for obstetrics, surgery, and dentistry. Success depends upon the ability of the patient to concentrate upon his motivation, his ability to react spontaneously, and his potential for detachment.

The medical literature contains many reports of surgery performed with hypnosis as the sole anesthetic, of relief provided from pain in injury or during childbirth. For chronic pain, said Dr. Finer, the picture is much more variable. There have been

[*] M.B.B.S., M.D., F.F.A.R.V.S., D.A., Associate Professor in Anesthesiology and Intensive Care, University of Uppsala, Sweden.
[2] "Clinical Use of Hypnosis in Pain Management," in press.

reports indicating complete pain relief, but there have also been many in which relief was not complete.

What has been achieved in some cases resembles the results of operant conditioning. It may reduce the suffering from an unbearable to a bearable level, enabling the patient to live and function when he had previously been unable to tolerate the pain.

Dr. Herbert Spiegel, who is Associate Professor of Psychiatry at Columbia University's College of Physicians and Surgeons, is a practicing psychiatrist in New York. His practice inevitably brings him people who are hurting. He has found hypnotism a practical tool, using it for such widely diverse objectives as curing migraine headaches or helping a patient to stop smoking.

Dr. Spiegel outlines three basic propositions to help explain the hypnotic phenomenon.

First, *alterations of awareness occur almost constantly*. The broadest and most obvious of these are the sleeping and waking rhythms of life. But in addition there are constant variations in awareness as we shift our attention from events going on at the fringes of our perception to concentrate on a central subject, or from scanning the entire stage before us to spotting fragmented experiences like momentary close-ups of passing events. Work has been done in this area of fragmentation experience by deliberately altering and reducing sensory input, to show how our awareness is in a constant state of change.

Second, *hypnotic phenomena occur whether they are identified as such or not*. There are a number of illustrations of such dissociated or hypnotic-like states quite familiar to us.

One is sleepwalking. People are known to get up from sleep, usually during or after a dream, walk around, even perform rather complicated acts without actually being awake.

Another is daydreaming, wherein a person can drift off into reverie which becomes so real that he loses all awareness of the actual world around him. The imagery in this moment of fantasy is actually the result of intense, focused concentration.

More extreme yet is a kind of fugue state in which some people experience a loss of time and place and, even when they come back from this dissociation, are unable to recall anything about the time warp they have just been through.

Still another experience has nothing to do with dissociation but is conscious voluntary concentration so intense that the individual blocks out everything around him and becomes completely oblivious to all the normal stimuli coming at him from every direction in his environment. This can take place during work, or it can take place in a theater where the spectator is so riveted by the drama on the stage that he becomes part of it, losing his surroundings and even his identity. Only when the curtain comes down does he realize again that he is sitting in a theater surrounded by other people, not part of the onstage action.

People in love can concentrate on one another to the point where they are oblivious to everyone and everything around them, so that they do not hear direct questions addressed to them or see events taking place directly in front of them.

There are literally dozens of such examples. Dr. Spiegel recalls an episode from *Shadows in the Grass*, a book about South Africa by Isak Dinesen, in which she describes an accident that happened to one of her native plantation workers. A tree he was cutting down fell on his leg, pinning him to the ground in intense pain. She sent for a car to take him to the hospital, but meanwhile she sat down on the ground, took his head in her lap, and tried to quiet him.

The man begged her to give him something to ease his pain. She had no drugs, but found some sugar cubes in her pockets and gave him one, telling him this would make him feel better. He sucked on the sugar cube and said it helped the pain. But when they were all gone he became anguished again. Looking for something else in her pockets she came across a letter. It happened to be from the King of Denmark, thanking her for the gift of a lion skin.

She told him this was powerful medicine because it came from a king, and she gave it to him to hold. He took the letter and relaxed, and said the pain was better. And he held the letter all the way to the hospital.

By the time he was released from the hospital the letter had become a talisman. A leather case was made for it to protect it from wearing out, because natives came from all the surrounding territory to cure their hurts by touching it.

Of course an exactly similar phenomenon can be seen in the grotto at Lourdes, or the shrine at St. Anne de Beaupré near Quebec, where hundreds of crutches hang on the walls as a testimonial to the people who came with them and left without them.

One curious thing about this suggestibility phenomenon is that it is not a one-way street, dependent only upon the patient. Dr. Beecher made a discovery in doing a surgical procedure for relieving the pain of angina pectoris, which consisted of tying off some of the arteries of the chest cage. When this operation was performed by a surgeon who was enthusiastic about the prospects of success, the rate of successful results was fifteen times better than when done by a surgeon who was skeptical about the results. A similar situation was found in operations for gastric ulcer.

Says Dr. Spiegel, "Beecher also revived a thesis about pain that Marshall and Strong developed in the late nineteenth century, in which they proposed that there is a physical stimulus to pain as one component, but by far the outstanding aspect of pain experience is the reactivity, or the processing component. If that can be channelized, the overall experience that we call pain can be appreciably modified." [3]

We are talking about hypnosis, but to be accurate it must be emphasized that none of the foregoing illustrations is really hypnosis. They are all examples of *altered awareness* and *dissociation,* with increased focal attention to some aspect of the particular situation. The *unique* feature of hypnosis is that it is deliberately set in motion and controlled by the hypnotist, taking full advantage of the responsiveness of the subject.

Dr. Spiegel calls it the "relative abandonment of executive control into a more-or-less regressed dissociated state. It is actively instigated and knowingly enhanced by the hypnotist and structured for goal achievement. . . . Hypnosis is only hypnosis when the hypnotist is knowingly in charge."

The third basic proposition of hypnosis is that nothing is achieved in therapy with hypnosis that cannot also be achieved without hypnosis. Then why use it? Because it can greatly shorten the time needed for therapy.

In pain, or in some stress conditions, time can be a very important factor. Take, as a rather extreme example, a suicide-prone neurotic. It is vital to get at the causes of his despair as quickly as possible rather than to run the risk of a suicide attempt during the ordinary slow-moving therapy. Hypnosis may be able to deal with the problem in a single session as against weeks or months

[3] "The Spectrum of Hypnotic and Non-Hypnotic Phenomena," *The American Journal of Clinical Hypnosis,* Vol. 6, July 1963, pp. 1-5.

of ordinary therapy, during which time there might always be the danger of another suicide attempt.

How effective is hypnosis? The following case histories are from Dr. Spiegel's records and are not offered as conclusive proof of miraculous effectiveness, but as examples of operating potential.

Case 1. The patient, a twenty-eight-year-old male, had intense and constant pain in his back and leg due to an inoperable and spreading carcinoma of the spine. Drugs had become ineffective and his surgeon, Dr. A, was planning a cordotomy for pain relief. Dr. B, also on the case, had meanwhile determined that the patient was hypnotizable and shortly taught him to control the pain by hypno-anesthesia. The patient was then able to walk the hospital corridor, something he had been unable to do for some time, to the surprise of his wife and nurse. Dr. A then arrived, learned what had happened, and became angry. He told the patient that hypnosis was nonsense, that pain could not be treated by pretending it was imaginary, that his pain was real, and that the cordotomy would be done as scheduled. The patient collapsed, his pain returned, and he could no longer walk.

Case 2. The patient, a twenty-six-year-old female, had Hodgkin's disease. Following surgery she had developed severe abdominal pain and was on a rising dosage of Demerol. Her life expectancy was several years and narcotic addiction was an obvious problem. Dr. C attempted hypnosis and it was successful enough to permit discontinuance of all drugs for pain.

Dr. C turned over daily reinforcement of the hypnotic anesthesia to the resident, Dr. D, who was at the time undergoing analysis as part of his own training. In the course of one of Dr. D's sessions with his analyst, he reported the interesting circumstance that he was helping a patient to remain pain-free without medication. The analyst became disturbed and instantly ordered him to stop using an unconventional technique while he was in the midst of his own analysis.

Dr. D then faced the dilemma of either disobeying or abandoning his patient. He decided to stall for a couple of days until he could shift his patient to another physician. The next day, however, he was unable to induce the patient to achieve the trance state, presumably because she picked up his own uncertainty. Her pain returned and she had to be given Demerol again.

The next day Dr. C returned, took over the patient, and was able to help her achieve her deep trance state. The pain was again banished and she was able to give up the narcotic.

Case 3. The patient, a thirty-four-year-old female, had severe chest pain, coughed up bloody sputum, and was subject to nausea and vomiting. She was unable to swallow and could not therefore eat or drink, so she was hospitalized and put on intravenous feeding. She had had three previous episodes of chest pain and cough, but these earlier spells had been without the nausea and vomiting.

After the third incident, her physician, Dr. E, had performed an operation which he guaranteed would prevent recurrence. Thus, when the fourth attack of chest pain and bloody cough began some six months after the operation, the frightened woman accused Dr. E of incompetence, deception, and betrayal. The doctor became upset, and his anxiety was picked up by the patient, whereupon nausea and vomiting began.

Dr. F was called in, to be told by a now thoroughly alarmed Dr. E that he considered the case so critical as to be terminal, meaning that he did not expect the patient to survive. Dr. F was able to induce the patient to enter a hypnotic state in which she became relaxed, her chest felt numb rather than wracked with pain, and the nausea diminished. She was able to drink some orange juice and the next day was able to eat and retain her food. On the following day she went home.

Case 4. The patient, a forty-year-old housewife, had suffered hysterical convulsive seizures lasting ten minutes, for a year and a half. These seizures occurred as often as eight to twelve times a day, sometimes during sleep. She had total amnesia about them and remembered nothing when they were over. Fortunately she was never hurt during any of these spells.

Neurological examination ruled out epilepsy. Her physician, Dr. G, tried the usual tranquilizer and sedative drugs, but they did not control or end the seizures. Dr. G told her there were only two choices, to live with the condition, or to be hospitalized.

The patient then went to another physician, Dr. H, who found that the seizures could be induced in the hypnotic state. The patient was taught to voluntarily activate a seizure at a learned signal. She was then taught that in the same way that she could produce a seizure, she could stop one. Her skill at control progressed to the point where in a few weeks she was able to abort an approaching seizure by triggering a token seizure which lasted only about five seconds.

Her ability to assert control restored her confidence and reintroduced her to a normal way of life without the constant fear of an impending seizure. She was able to function competently again as wife and mother without the watchful supervision of other members of the family. No insight therapy was required. The cause of mechanism of the seizures was not revealed. But their constant menace was removed, and she was offered the opportunity of a normal life with her self-esteem restored.

Now, please note that there is a common factor in all four cases. In none has the hypnotist attempted to dig out the root cause of the illness. Hypnosis has only removed the symptoms. From the medical standpoint this brings up the question: is the removal of symptoms dangerous when the root cause of the condition is untouched?

Obviously there are situations in which symptom removal can be dangerous. The patient who closes his eyes to a serious organic illness by masking symptoms is merely postponing for a while the day of reckoning. But as we have already seen, there are other situations in which pain is present without organic illness or structural damage.

There are physicians, Dr. Spiegel points out, who are convinced that alleviation of psychiatric symptoms is dangerous because new or worse symptoms are sure to follow. Out of this fear, as in some of the above cases, they would actually deny the patient an unconventional treatment that might help.

"The prevalence of this belief," says Dr. Spiegel, "is especially ironic because medicine has traditionally resorted to symptom alleviation as a major treatment procedure. It is obvious that although the elimination of causative disease agents or core factors is desirable ideally, we cannot in fact easily identify and circumscribe the core factors of complex disabling processes. Furthermore, since the notion of basic causes for psychiatric illness remains a hypothetical concept, and therefore ambiguous and clinically elusive, treatment cannot really resolve such core or basic factors." [4]

Against the belief that removing symptoms merely bottles up a kind of psychic energy that must pop out in new symptoms elsewhere, Dr. Spiegel proposes another suggestion. This is that learning to master a disabling symptom generates a kind of momentum which leads to mastery in other areas. Essential to the whole question is *the crucial role of expectancy in the therapeutic atmosphere*—that is, the patient's own expectations about treatment and/or his response to the doctor's expectations."

The same patients who respond well to suggestion or to placebos may lose ground as they pick up some indication of a doctor's pessimism or anxiety. Not all patients are quite such weathervanes and many recover as much in spite of the doctor as because of him. But there is a general agreement that the element of hope plays a very large role in recovery and that communication of hope from the therapist to the patient is of definite benefit.

Is symptom removal dangerous? The question is pretty much on the order of "Have you stopped beating your wife?" The correct answer is "When?" Surely in benign chronic pain, where the symptom is the disease itself, symptom removal is of the essence. It needs to be done with skill and compassion, and it needs to be done in full understanding of the curious fact that removing a symptom may leave a void in the patient's life. Therefore the therapist must be sure that the patient can stand having the symptom removed.

Can a patient live without the pain that has become a way of life for him? He can, if he is taught to fill the void with activity worth more than pain-behavior.

[4] "Is Symptom Removal Dangerous?" *American Journal of Psychiatry,* Vol. 123, April 1967, p. 10.

Chapter 14

ACUPUNCTURE

Acupuncture is based on the fact that stimulation of the skin has an effect on the internal organs and other parts of the body, a relatively simple reflex whose therapeutic application is largely ignored in the West.

FELIX MANN, M.B.[1]

The near-superstitious awe with which the American public greeted reports of miraculous cures through acupuncture was in the main viewed with caution by Western physicians. A few have made pilgrimages to Peking and returned filled with enthusiasm, but other observers have been much more reserved and others are openly skeptical.

American physicians, in fact, seem divided between those who urge trials of acupuncture and those who label it hypnosis with gadgetry. The literature on acupuncture is already extensive, not even counting the ancient Chinese writings.

In fact the controversy is not confined to Western doctors alone. It has been going on in China itself for at least a hundred years, with the Chinese divided between their traditional medicine and a need to import the new Western techniques.

As folklore therapy, acupuncture is at least 3,000 years old. Its use to control pain, and as analgesia in surgery, dates back

[1] *Acupuncture; the Ancient Chinese Art of Healing and How It Works Scientifically,* revised edn., Vintage Books, New York, 1973.

only a few years, to the Communist revolution, when modern China began to break out of much of the traditional past.

Acupuncture is not even exclusively Chinese. The ancient Egyptians practiced some form of it; the Arabs utilized a kind of ear acupuncture using a hot iron; some Eskimo tribes apply a crude acupuncture using sharp-edged stones; a tribe in Brazil shoots small arrows at specific parts of the body through a blow-pipe. It remained for the Chinese to elaborate the incredibly complicated system or group of systems we now know, surrounding it with religious and mystical ritual so involved that it takes years to master, or even to understand.

Because human dissection was not allowed in China, tradi-tional Chinese doctors had no accurate idea of the human anat-omy; moreover they consistently identified parts of the body and the various diseases which afflict them with the universe and with certain spiritual or mystical forces operating within it.

In this Chinese mythology there are five elements: Wood, Fire, Earth, Metal (or Air), and Water. Everything on earth belongs to one or more of these five elements. A pentagon, or five-sided figure, can be drawn with one of the five elements at each corner. A line connecting each point is the "outer" line, described as the "creative" line. You can also draw lines inside the penta-gon, crossing the interior to connect the points from the inside. These lines are the "destructive" forces. Thus the litany:

Wood burns to create Fire, which leaves Earth as ash, out of which may be extracted Metal, which can be heated to become molten like Water, which is needed for plants to grow, which forms Wood. This is the outer line or creative cycle.

Wood can destroy Earth (plant roots break up soil and rocks), Earth destroys Water (water cannot seep through a clay pot), Water extinguishes Fire, Fire destroys Metal (by melting it), Metal destroys Wood (an axe cuts down a tree). These are the inner lines, or destructive forces.

Everything on earth, including man's internal organs, belongs to one or another of the five elements. There is another control-ling factor, the Yin and Yang, dual expressions of Qi (or Ch'i), the life force which flows along the meridians Ching Lo. All parts of the body are either Yin or Yang, all illnesses are either Yin or Yang, and all therapy is either Yin or Yang. Acupuncture needles are used to restore the balance of Yin and Yang or to resume the flow of Qi along the meridians where it may be blocked.

Everything that is Yin is passive, feminine, negative. Everything that is Yang is aggressive, positive, and masculine. These chauvinistic teams line up inside us like this:

Wood: Represents in Yin the liver, in Yang the gallbladder.
Fire: In Yin the heart, in Yang the small intestine.
Earth: The spleen in Yin, the stomach in Yang.
Metal: In Yin the lung, in Yang the large intestine.
Water: The kidney in Yin, the bladder in Yang.
Fire: In Yin the pericardium, in Yang the Triple Warmer.

The pericardium is the fibrous sac that surrounds the heart. The Triple Warmer or the "Three Burning Spaces" has yet to be isolated or identified. Even the Chinese are not clear about this elusive organ. Some describe the Triple Warmer as a kind of sewage system, others say it moves the vital fluids between the solid and hollow organs, and others describe it as the link between man and the universe.

Chinese writing has rhythm and power even in translation, as witness this from Su Wen in the traditional writings:

If there is a surplus of Qi, then control that which is already winning and antagonize that which is not winning; if there is a deficiency of Qi, then antagonize and regulate that which is not winning and bring out and antagonize that which is winning.

Or from the Nan Jing:

If a disease has empty evil, full evil, thief evil, minute evil and upright evil, how can they be distinguished? That which comes from behind is empty evil, that which comes from in front is full evil, that which comes from the not-winning is thief evil, that which comes from the winning is minute evil, and autogenous disease is upright evil.

If for some reason this is not completely clear, then peruse this explanation by Dr. Felix Mann, the renowned English authority on acupuncture:

"The quotation indicates the various paths taken by 'invading disease evils.' Empty evil coming from behind is a mother disease affecting the son, as for instance a liver disease which is transmitted to the heart. Full evil coming from in front is a son disease going back to the mother, like a disease of the spleen which is transmitted to the heart. Thief evil coming from the not-winning can be illustrated by a liver disease being transmitted to the spleen, and minute evil coming from the winning, by a lung disease transmitted to the heart. Upright evil is an autogenous heart disease, originating in the heart, and is not transmitted to any other organ." [2]

Understandably, this kind of ritual turned off many Western physicians who might otherwise have been interested. After all, acupuncture has been around for a long time and, if as successful as claimed, certainly warranted a long hard look by Western science. The claims made for cures of disease concern us less here than the use of acupuncture for the control of pain, its more modern usage.

With the coming of the Communist regime in China a huge effort began to clean up the maze of small, feudal, corrupt governments such as they were, and to provide among other services, some kind of medical care system. It was obviously impossible to mount a crash program to train students in Western medicine; equipment was lacking and there was a block of ingrained tradition and inertia to be overcome. Chairman Mao announced, "Chinese medicine and pharmacology are a great treasure house; efforts should be made to explore them and raise them to a higher level."

The obvious strategy was to combine the old and the new, to set up short training courses for paramedics—the barefoot doctors—and to use all existing medical personnel, whatever their training had been.

It was this collaboration that resulted in the use of acupuncture for general anesthesia, a use not common until then. Traditionally, acupuncture practitioners were opposed to surgery, but apparently have been swept up, despite themselves, in the modernization movement.

Today, instead of talking about meridians, or peripheral tubes, they are considering the possibility that their needles are influencing peripheral nerves, and in an attempt to explain how acupuncture works, are edging closer to the wholly Western Melzack-Wall gate theory.

Dr. H. Jack Geiger was a member of an eleven-man American

[2] *Acupuncture.*

medical team that spent twenty-two days in China and reported, in a series of articles for *Medical World News,* his impressions of Chinese medicine.

At the Institute of Physiology in Shanghai a research team headed by Professor Chang Hsiang Tung, a neurophysiologist who studied at Yale and returned to China in the fifties, is investigating the use of acupuncture in analgesia.

Professor Chang told Dr. Geiger, "We believe that the analgesic effect of acupuncture is a central nervous system effect, the result of interaction of different afferent impulses, some from the site of acupuncture, others from the site of pain. These two sets of impulses interact on each other at different levels of the CNS—in the spinal cord as we have shown, and in the thalamus, which is probably the most important site." [3]

There could hardly be a better description of the Melzak-Wall gate theory, which we have now encountered in several different disciplines.

The Chinese, Dr. Geiger says, believe that acupuncture alters the patient's perception of pain by a blocking action in the CNS which is achieved without the depressant effect of drugs or loss of consciousness. Anesthesia is produced either by the use of needles or of deep massage, for both the Chinese and Japanese have discovered that simple pressure will often serve as well as needles. According to Dr. Tsung O. Cheng,* an American physician born in China, who returned for a visit in 1972, injections of distilled water are also used. [4]

Although hundreds of acupuncture points are clearly identified on the ancient charts and models, the number of needles used has been declining. One Chinese surgeon told Dr. Geiger that when they first began using acupuncture for analgesia they might have used forty needles in all four limbs, with four acupuncturists and a "conductor" to orchestrate the entire performance. "Even if it worked," he said, "who needed it? You couldn't get close to the table." Gradually the number of needles was

[3] "How Acupuncture Anesthetizes: The Chinese Explanation," *Medical World News,* Vol. 14, July 13, 1973, pp. 51-61.
* Professor of Medicine, George Washington School of Medicine, Washington, D.C.; Associate Director, Division of Cardiology.
[4] "Medicine in Modern China," *Journal of the American Geriatrics Society,* Vol. 21, No. 7, July 1973, pp. 289-296.

reduced to twenty, then to ten, then to a few, to one or now even none.

What is not generally realized in the West is that the great majority of surgical operations in China are done with conventional chemical anesthesia—only 20 or 30 percent are done with acupuncture. The patient is given free choice as to which he selects. Moreover, even if they choose acupuncture, most patients are given preoperative doses of morphine or Demerol in any case. After the operation, pain is managed both with drugs and additional acupuncture.

Four or five days are given to preparation—one might say psychological conditioning—of the patient, with reassurance and instruction as to what is going to happen. And if the patient still appears nervous or anxious, conventional anesthesia is used —no chances are taken with acupuncture and a fully awake patient.

All of this may strongly suggest hypnosis, a theory the Chinese strongly reject. As Dr. Geiger says, "The anesthetic effect is *not* due to any kind of hypnosis, unless one is willing to accept the unlikely proposition that horses, mules, cats, rats, rabbits, and human infants are susceptible to hypnosis, whether by standard techniques or by acupuncture needling."

Nevertheless no less an authority than Professor Pat Wall, co-author of the Melzack-Wall gate theory, says bluntly that he considers acupuncture "an effective use of hypnosis."

The effectiveness of any therapeutic method, says Professor Wall, is very difficult to test. Even in double-blind tests with morphine, 80 percent of the patients said they had relief from pain, but 60 percent gained the same relief from a placebo. Tests for the effectiveness of acupuncture have not been done. It is his guess that if those tests are carried out, it will be found that acupuncture does not "generate the specifically pain-inhibiting barrage for which I was looking." [5]

If acupuncture does prove to be hypnosis, this would not diminish its usefulness, but it would at least remove the mysticism surrounding it. "We must remember," says Professor Wall, "the cultural tradition of the (Chinese) patient, who comes not only from a society proud of its stoicism in the face of suffering, but

[5] "An Eye on the Needle," *New Scientist,* Vol. 55, July 1972, pp. 129-31.

one in which acupuncture has been accepted for millennia as powerful medicine."

The Chinese patient's conditioning toward acupuncture is not only of long standing, but is now greatly reinforced by the flood of publicity it has had, plus the surge of national pride, fanned by the flattering attention of visiting foreign doctors and professors.

The prolonged instruction and conditioning which precede any use of acupuncture for surgery supports the suspicion that, intentionally or not, these patients are undergoing a strong form of suggestion. Professor Wall believes the key to this procedure lies in the realization that acupuncture is not used on children, although certainly their brains are fully functioning by the age of five.

In a state of hypnosis, the patient yields control to the hypnotist, including decisions about the relevancy of his behavior. Reaction to pain (and tissue damage) is also a form of behavior, as we have seen, and is controllable by hypnosis. Children, certainly, are suggestible, but not in this complicated transfer of responsibility. They do not react to placebos. And they have not yet learned that the needle and syringe bring relief from pain, or in the case of Chinese children that the acupuncture needle works the same miracle. And, if they do not believe it will work, it does not work. Yet Dr. Cheng says that finger-pressing acupuncture is good anesthesia for children who are having dental work done.

It is argued that animals respond to acupuncture, therefore something other than hypnotism must be operating in their case. Both Professor Wall and Dr. Spiegel point out that animals can easily be hypnotized by simple restraint. There is a difference between sophisticated hypnosis which uses verbal persuasion and "animal hypnotism."

A child who is wrapped up tightly will become much more quiet than a child left free. This, says Professor Wall, is the basis of the worldwide practice of "swaddling." Similarly, many animals (and some adult humans), if restrained, pass into a trancelike state during which minor surgery can be performed with no pain reaction.

This is the state, Professor Wall believes, which is induced in some of the Chinese demonstrations of acupuncture on animals.

Even in human adults, hypnotists try to get their patients into a "still reaction" before going into the more sophisticated phase of verbal persuasion. While only 7 percent of Americans or British can be hypnotized easily, 60 percent are placebo reactors who will perform reliably when given something they believe to be a narcotic.

It is thus possible, he argues, that the Chinese patient, given a choice and himself selecting acupuncture, and having been preconditioned all his life to believe in it, is simply going to have a much higher rate of response than an unconditioned American.

Yet, with all that, some Chinese still do not respond to acupuncture anesthesia, which makes Professor Wall the more likely to believe that it is a highly personal form of therapy like hypnosis, rather than an effect common to everybody, like inhaling ether or taking a barbiturate.

During his trip to China, Dr. E. Grey Dimond discussed the hypnosis theory with Dr. Chen Tseg-Ming, Chief of Anesthesia at the Kwangtung Provincial People's Hospital in Canton. Dr. Chen is a Western-trained anesthetist.

"Did he believe there was any element of hypnotism or autosuggestion involved? He laughed and said, 'Obviously not.' The method was being used in every hospital in China by literally thousands of physicians and upon hundreds of thousands of patients. Did we think everyone was hypnotized? If a patient with a severe fracture came to the emergency room, acupuncture anesthesia was routinely used, as they had found a much-decreased incidence of shock. Such patients had no prior discussion with the anesthetist, thus there was no opportunity for autosuggestion." [6]

Professor Wall might argue here that the element of preconditioning and the willingness to believe are being overlooked. It was the dependability of the general anesthetic which made surgeons prefer it over hypnosis or other systems which have long been available. Admittedly there is a certain amount of risk in using general anesthesia, and for this reason local anesthetics are used wherever possible, which is why anesthetists are interested in acupuncture.

Manipulating the needles by electric current is part of the

[6] "Acupuncture Anesthesia," *Journal of the American Medical Association*, Vol. 218, No. 10, December 6, 1971, pp. 1558-63.

modernization of the ancient art. It strongly suggests operation of the gate theory—if you stimulate a nerve, you raise the pain threshold by closing the gate in the spinal cord. It may be, therefore, that by using electric current, acupuncture is moving from a kind of general hypnosis to local stimulation which produces local analgesia.

The more one examines it, the more fascinating becomes the proposed link between acupuncture and hypnosis. Dr. William S. Kroger, Executive Director of the Institute for Comprehensive Medicine, Beverly Hills, California, points out the similarities between patient preparation for surgery under hypnosis and under acupuncture:

"Rehearsal of the entire surgical procedure, preoperatively, blocks the neurophysiological pathways involved in pain transmission. Thus receptions in the higher brain centers, when they are experientially conditioned under autogenic training or autohypnosis, protect the patient from surprise, apprehension, fear and tension, and raise the pain threshold. Often, with highly motivated patients, hypnotic induction was not required when autogenic training was employed." [7]

Dr. Kroger recalls that the potency of this training was brought home to him by the fact that the only time a patient complained of pain was when the towel clips touched the skin of the abdomen before any incision was made. This happened to be the only detail left out of the rehearsal, and indicates how precise the conditioned response can be.

Similarly, at the Friendship Hospital in Peking, patients go through several days of rehearsal before surgery, with the surgeons carefully explaining everything they are going to do. The patient is shown how the operation will be done, what the acupuncturist will do, and what effect the needles should have. The patient is encouraged to talk to others who already have had surgery with acupuncture. And finally, if he wishes, the patient can take home some acupuncture needles to experiment with by himself.

This "preparation" is reminiscent of the preparation employed in natural childbirth, one of the most outstanding forms of pain

---

[7] "Acupuncture Analgesia: Its Explanation by Conditioning Theory, Autogenic Training, and Hypnosis." Read at the 126th Annual Meeting of the American Psychiatric Association, Honolulu, May 7-11, 1973.

156 The Conquest of Pain

control and of training for no-drug birth. In natural childbirth other factors come into the picture—breathing and muscle control. But removing fear of the unknown through preparation for surgery and rehabilitation is used in a number of fields, especially with heart-attack victims.

As a psychiatrist, Dr. Spiegel became interested in what he suspected might be a correlation between hypnotism and acupuncture, and began collecting cases of people who did not respond to either. He reported his early findings to Dr. Ronald Katz, then chief anesthesiologist at Columbia's College of Physicians and Surgeons. Dr. Katz began to investigate this phenomenon himself.

In May 1973, Dr. Katz summarized his collaboration with Dr. Spiegel in a paper delivered at the Seattle symposium on pain.

"Preliminary results," said Dr. Katz, "suggest a correlation (between susceptibility to hypnosis and responsiveness to acupuncture analgesia), but this by no means indicates a cause and effect." However, it did seem to indicate that they are parallel processes.

There are some differences. Under hypnosis the patient shows "a narrow band of focused inner attention," which is the trance state. This is not present during acupuncture and the patient can talk easily and naturally with the physician.

Said Dr. Katz, "We have found it possible to carry out surgical procedures with acupuncture as the sole anesthetic. Acute and chronic pain have also been relieved by acupuncture. However, it is our belief that acupuncture is no panacea and that there is insufficient data to determine its relative effectiveness as compared with other therapeutic regimes. The long-term effectiveness of acupuncture in pain relief is also not yet known."

Dr. John W. C. Fox, Assistant Professor of Anesthesiology at New York's Downstate Medical Center, with his wife Elisabeth who is also an anesthesiologist, uses acupuncture under three specific conditions: for minor surgery only; for patients in whom an orthodox medical diagnosis has been established with pain a disabling feature and for whom conventional techniques fail to provide relief; and for neurophysiologic research in medical personnel volunteers.

Dr. Fox is undisturbed by the possibility that acupuncture and hypnotism may be similar or identical.

"The purpose of medicine," he says, "is to improve performance, relieve suffering, and restore the patient toward normalcy, whatever you want to define normal as being. The beauty of acupuncture, as I see it, is that we are not giving any drugs, we are not poisoning the patient, we are not going to have any side effects. There must be some side effects, there undoubtedly can be, besides the obvious ones if you don't sterilize the needles or wipe off the skin."

In his experience, says Dr. Fox, acupuncture will relieve pain —temporarily. But it is far from a cure-all, and its mode of action is unknown.

Dr. Kroger says, "From the welter of mutually contradictory theories and speculations having low predictive value, it is obvious that acupunctural analgesia has not been satisfactorily explained by the Melzack-Wall skin-sensory gating mechanism, or by any other theory. I stated that acupunctural anesthesia works largely by 'suggestion in slow motion—hypnosis.'"

He quotes Professor Wall from "An Eye on the Needle": "My own belief is that in this context [anesthesia], acupuncture is an effective use of hypnosis. This in no way dismisses or diminishes the value of acupuncture, but it does place it in a class of phenomena with which we are partly familiar."

Professor Wall continues: "To put this in its historical perspective, we should remember that major surgery under mesmerism was widely practiced in the London teaching hospitals two hundred years ago until it was displaced by ether and then chloroform general anesthesia. These mesmerized patients, like the ones under acupuncture, were conscious and talking during the operation, aware of events around them, but they were not in pain and did not show reflex responses to the cuts being made. They were not generally anesthetized because they could sense events on other parts of their body except where they were directed to feel no pain."

There are other points of view. Dr. Chapman, of Seattle's Pain Clinic, says, "I've worked with both hypnosis and acupuncture and I would never dismiss either of them. I wouldn't combine them as the same phenomenon, but I think that the two phenomena may have a common root—a common explanation. I wouldn't say acupuncture is just hypnosis. We don't understand hypnosis and why label one mystery as another?"

Dr. Crue, of the City of Hope, says, "We're convinced—I am personally—that most of acupuncture is conditioning and due to psychological suggestion—the placebo effect—so we're not doing needle acupuncture the Chinese way. When we do acupuncture we use electric current and we do it transcutaneously. We long ago gave up using needles.

"Hypnosis and acupuncture are not the same but they are very, very similar. They work at a different level, but I'm convinced that they are probably very similar neurophysiologically. If you are going to use acupuncture for input it doesn't really matter whether you put electric current in the needle through the skin, put pressure on, burn and use heat—moxibustion on the surface—place the needles through tubes, or twirl them. You can do it different ways and I don't think it really makes a bit of difference. It's the input stimuli into this person's central nervous system, which is being further conditioned, that is the important factor. The psychological set of that individual is also very important.

"We've done the same thing in this country. When your grandmother put a mustard plaster on your chest it was pretty effective. It burned so you forgot your cough in a hurry, and I'm old enough to remember it."

Acupuncture, says Dr. Crue, must be considered as it relates to three different applications. First, there is the treatment of chronic diseases like arthritis or diabetes, for which he feels it is not to be taken seriously. "You don't find many reputable neurophysiologists or M.D.'s in this country talking about acupuncture for the treatment of diabetes."

Second, it is used in the treatment of the chronic pain syndrome. The third use for acupuncture is in anesthesia. Apparently it is most successful in the last.

"Let me give you two examples that I think make a point. There's a lady in this hospital who is full of cancer. She's had multiple operations. She's had a mastectomy; her spine has collapsed; she can hardly move her legs; when she does move, it grinds and hurts because she's got a pathological fracture of the hip. When the nurses turn her bed, they just try to ease her over to change the sheets, but she screams in pain. It's pretty horrible. There's never been a patient, I think you could say, who had more reason to hurt.

"We explained to her that we were going to put this electric current on her neck. We strapped on a plate the way we do, hooked it up to a fancy-looking box, set it up where she could see it, and told her we didn't know whether or not it would work. We weren't promising a thing."

This gadget was the transcutaneous stimulator, City of Hope's candidate for acupuncture.

"We went back the next morning and found that she'd slept right through the night for the first time. She hadn't awakened once, she hadn't asked for morphine. She was so happy she was radiant. I can't describe to you how much better she was—there's only one little point you ought to know. We hadn't plugged it into the electric wall outlet.

"The second case is an example of how sophisticated you can get in making areas anesthetic. I had a lab technician who had worked with me for fourteen years, mostly with the microscope, on tissue culture. She had nothing to do with pain, and she doesn't know much about electricity either. But she had been with me a long time and she had faith in me—or in what we're trying to do.

"She knew that across the hall from her lab we were working with electric current, trying to make people numb, trying to see if we could take pain away.

"I called her and said, 'I'd like you to try this. We've tried it ourselves and it's safe. Let's be our own guinea pigs, if you are willing. We're going to put this on your neck and run a current through it.'

"Then I dropped a key phrase. I knew that she knew her anatomy. I said, 'I want to see what effect passing a current through here will have on sensation in the trigeminal region.'

"She had no pain in this area; she was perfectly normal. But she knows exactly where the trigeminal area is. And she became absolutely anesthetic in both sides of her face, right down to her neck and the lower half of the ear. We tried her with pins. You could take a sterile hypo needle and put it right through the skin with no pain.

"We didn't hypnotize her, but we used suggestion. That's what acupuncture is. You don't have to go into a trance state. Right now there is no proof that acupuncture works in the human for chronic pain or for anesthesia better than suggestion. This is what these two cases mean to me. You can take normal people, or pain patients, and by suggestion do exactly the same thing."

Dr. Richard Black, coordinator of the Seattle Pain Clinic, agrees with Dr. Crue that acupuncture is not hypnotism, but that suggestion probably plays a large part. "What is hypnotism and what is suggestion, and where do you draw the line? I think there are graded changes there, I don't think there is a line to be drawn."

Dr. Mann's book, *Acupuncture,* carries the subtitle *The Ancient Chinese Art of Healing and How It Works Scientifically.* Although Dr. Mann demolishes most of the mysticism surrounding Yin and Yang, the five elements, and the meridians, he retained his enthusiasm for acupuncture right up to the 1973 revised edition of the book.

His conclusions, he says, "might give the reader the impression that there is little left to acupuncture, for I have demolished practically the whole of the traditional theoretical framework. This is far from being the case, for I practice acupuncture exclusively about 90 percent of my time, and I would not do so if I did not achieve better results than in practicing Western medicine in the appropriate type of disease or dysfunction. There are, of course, many diseases where Western medicine is better than acupuncture."

On July 14, 1973, Dr. Mann reported on a study of pain in *The Lancet,* an influential British medical journal.[8] The paper took account of some of the current controversy.

His four collaborators had never seen acupuncture in action before the summer of 1972, and admitted to being skeptical about it. For their study, eighteen patients with intractable pain were treated. All had proved resistant to orthodox procedures.

The patients suffered from the now-familiar list of injuries or disease: operations for lumbar disk protrusion, post-herpetic neuralgia, carcinoma, and so on, all conditions of severe and stubborn pain.

Of the eighteen people, ten experienced relief with acupuncture treatment ranging from partial to total; eight had no relief, or improvement so slight as to suggest the patient was merely trying to encourage the doctors.

[8] Felix Mann et al., "Treatment of Intractable Pain by Acupuncture," Vol. 2, pp. 57-60.

Predicting results with acupuncture, said the authors, was not possible, but they add, "except that, like hypnosis, acupuncture is considerably less effective in cases which are mainly functional." This is a curious statement, one would expect the exact opposite to be true.

The report also notes that, at the pain symposium in Seattle, the suggestion was made that the proportion of patients helped by acupuncture was about the same as those aided by placebo, and referred to the Katz paper suggesting a correlation between patients susceptible to acupuncture and hypnotism. "However," said the report, "it was generally felt that a neurophysiological basis (for acupuncture) must be positively disproved before it can be excluded. It appears, moreover, that in practiced hands, the relief rate in acupuncture is higher than that from either placebo reaction or hypnosis."

A month later *The Lancet* published a paper on acupuncture by Dr. G. M. Bull,[9] who is associated with the Medical Research Council Clinical Research Centre at Harrow, Middlesex, England. In this study, Dr. Bull examined the "two hypotheses currently favored to explain how acupuncture might induce anesthesia. The one is hypnotism and the other is the so-called Gate Hypothesis of Melzack and Wall."

Dr. Bull suggested that neither theory accounted for the fact that it seemed to be necessary for acupuncture needles to be vibrated or rotated, either manually or by electricity. And he proposed a new theory to explain how acupuncture works. His theory was that the rhythmic stimulation caused areas of the cerebral cortex to become "locked on" to the rhythm and so busy with it that they simply did not respond to other stimuli in their normal manner.

This sounds like distraction, which we have seen in other forms. There have been recent reports that Chinese theorists also are considering that acupuncture may act as a distraction rather than as a pain block. But Dr. Bull remarked that his hypothesis was not inconsistent with a participation of some hypnotic effects, adding, "The mechanism of hypnosis has never been adequately explained."

Dr. Mann replied to Dr. Bull's paper a few weeks later with

9 "Acupuncture Anesthesia," Vol. 2, August 25, 1973, pp. 417-18.

a letter to *The Lancet.*[10] This new hypothesis, he said, was interesting insofar as it coincided with many of the facts recorded in acupuncture analgesia, but many of these facts were open to doubt. He then went on to outline a surprising modification of his long-standing enthusiasm for acupuncture.

Having performed acupuncture anesthesia on more than 100 occasions, he said, he has concluded that it works well in only about 10 percent of cases. In 65 percent the anesthesia was "mild and patchy" and in the remaining 25 percent there was no effect or nearly no effect. Some of the patients in that mid-zone of 65 percent could be anesthetized "if the stimulus was increased to what for a Westerner are torture levels."

This says something very interesting. Do the Chinese withstand a rate of stimulation so high that it would be unbearable to a Westerner because they have been preconditioned? Perhaps for generations? And if so, what does this suggest?

The 10 percent of cases in which acupuncture worked well, Dr. Mann said, were not responding to a hypnotic phenomenon because the analgesia will take place in the correct area even if the patient is told it will happen somewhere else.

Acupuncture anesthesia, he now believes, is more like dental anesthesia by white sound, which, as we have already noted, requires *both* the sound *and* suggestion to work. Either by itself will not do.

Dr. Bull's rhythm theory, Dr. Mann suggests, does not fully explain the acupuncture effect because the frequency of the stimulation is not important, but the size of the stimulus is. There appears to be a correlation between many of the acupuncture points and the peripheral nervous system, although this is purely theoretical since acupuncture points "exist no more than do the coordinates of a star."

All of this is bound to be upsetting to a great many acupuncture enthusiasts who are convinced of the authenticity of a thousand acupuncture points, each controlling a specific area of the body. But there is more upset to come.

Dr. Mann's letter went on to say that he knew of no reliable report in the West of acupuncture anesthesia being 90 percent effective as claimed. "There are many initial enthusiastic reports,

[10] "Acupuncture Anesthesia," Vol. 2, September 8, 1973, pp. 563-4.

including my own, which have mellowed with further experience. When I was subjected to acupuncture analgesia by Chinese doctors who had done several hundred operations by this means, it failed, even though it was tried on three occasions, and it failed likewise in a medical colleague who was present at the same time."

So great a change in acupuncture's most celebrated proponent is bound to have serious effects in American and British circles at least, if not in Chinese. But a fair conclusion from all this is that acupuncture may well work far better on the Chinese than on Westerners. And so the factor of suggestibility can hardly be ruled out. Studies are underway, some funded by the National Institutes of Health, another by the State of New York. And perhaps in the next few years some better answers may be forthcoming.

Chapter 15

BIOFEEDBACK

*The ultimate possibilities for man's self-control are nothing less
than the evolution of an entirely new culture where people can change
their mental and physical states as easily as switching
channels on a television set.*

MARVIN KARLINS, PH.D.
LEWIS M. ANDREWS, M. A.*

It would be extravagant to say that biofeedback burst upon the
public awareness with the same impact as acupuncture. Yet in
some circles its effect was comparable. *Medical World News*
reported in early 1973:[1]

The suggestion that asthma, epilepsy, hypertension, cardiac arrhyth-
mias, hemiplegia, migraine, tension headaches, torticollis spasms,
hyperkinesis, and functional disorders of many systems may all be
relieved by a single form of treatment sounds more like a nineteenth-
century pitch for snake oil than a true reflection of research in 1973.

The resemblance above to the many claims for acupuncture is
obvious, so also was the inevitable charge that biofeedback, like

---

* *Biofeedback*, J. B. Lippincott Co., Philadelphia, Pa., 1972. Marvin Karlins is Associate Professor of Psychology, City College of the City University
of New York. Lewis M. Andrews, A.B. in Psychology and M.A. in Com-
munications, has written two books on psychology.
[1] "Biofeedback in Action," Vol. 14, No. 10, March 9, 1973, pp. 47-60.

acupuncture, is merely another form of suggestion employing the placebo principle. Nevertheless, there are now a large number of serious scientists working with biofeedback and most of them say that despite undeniable elements of suggestion, there is also something different about it. It is a *learning* process.

The word "feedback" has earned permanent status in our language. It came out of the radio electronics research which began in the twenties. Dr. Norbert Wiener, the father of cybernetics, defined feedback as "a method of controlling a system by reinserting into it the results of past performance."

The statement contains dazzling potentialities, some of which have already been realized, viz., machines which correct their own errors. There is something disturbingly human about this and what is better, or worse, is that eventually it will lead to machines that can repair and rebuild themselves. When that happens, machines will be a clear step ahead of humans.

Add the prefix "bio" to feedback and you have a system which can monitor the signals coming from various organs of the body: heart, brain, muscles, stomach, and the rest. The organs under the control of the autonomic nervous system have always been considered outside voluntary control. Who could imagine controlling his heartbeat or blood pressure? Yet biofeedback training offers exactly this possibility. Using electronics, it tunes in on body functions and transposes them into a visible or audible signal that an individual can actually see or hear, and at once grasp what is going on in his own body. Once he can do that, the possibility of controlling those functions becomes a reality.

Biofeedback equipment can be improvised out of almost anything, but essentially it works out to an instrument that amplifies the electrical signals from the body to a readily detectable form: a light that flashes, a bell that rings, a pen that traces a course over a paper—anything of the sort.

In one hospital experiment, patients with premature ventricular contractions of the heart learned how to speed up or slow down their heartbeats. The instrument in this case was a cardiotachometer connected to a computer. Lying in bed, the patient could watch a kind of traffic light arrangement with three colors: red, green, and yellow. A green light meant "speed up," yellow meant "correct speed," and red meant "slow down."

Now there appears to be no logical reason why a patient lying in bed and watching traffic lights that indicate how fast his heart is beating should be able to change the speed. But in actual practice it turns out that he can. Not only were the patients in this and many other experiments able to control the rates of their hearts but they were able to smooth out the irregular beats from which some of them suffered.

Yoga adepts are able to demonstrate a similar ability to control bodily functions. The difference between yoga and biofeedback, however, is that yoga requires an enormous amount of self-discipline and skill, while biofeedback actually requires neither. The presence of the biofeedback machine establishes a learning environment which promotes the ability to control body functions far more easily and rapidly, with no real skill or self-discipline required.

Many of the stories coming out of biofeedback laboratories verge on the incredible. As early as the late sixties, Dr. Neal E. Miller, Professor of Physiological Psychology at Rockefeller University in New York, was reporting that he and his associates had taught laboratory rats to increase or decrease their heart rates, blood pressures, and intestinal functions through biofeedback responses that offered rewards for the right responses. They actually had cut it so fine that they were able to teach rats to make one ear blush without the other.

These results, said Dr. Miller, challenged the accepted belief that bodily functions in the autonomic nervous system were beyond conscious control.

Certainly the individual is not normally conscious of his blood pressure and hasn't much idea whether it is low, normal, or higher than it should be. Yet humans and rats can and have been taught to raise or lower this pressure.

At Harvard, Dr. Herbert Benson, Assistant Professor of Medicine, and Dr. David Shapiro, Assistant Professor of Psychology, worked with a group of seven patients, all of whom had higher than normal blood pressures. Six of the seven were able to lower systolic pressure by an average of 16.5 mm Hg.

Learning requires reinforcement, and the systems used to reinforce a correct response are sometimes amusing. With animals, reinforcement might consist of a reward such as food, or electrical stimulation of the pleasure center in the brain. Or, conversely, it might consist of avoidance of punishment, like an electric shock. With humans, the encouragement of seeing self-progress might be enough, but the Harvard psychologists added some trimmings. Not only did a change in the subject's blood pressure produce a light and a beep, but after every twenty beeps a slide was projected on a screen showing a soothing scenic land-scape and the total amount of money the patient had earned at a rate of five cents for every slide, plus the $5 paid for each session.

One theory for the ability to control blood pressure through biofeedback is advanced by Dr. William A. Love, Jr., director of the biofeedback research laboratory at Nova University in Fort Lauderdale, Florida. Using feedback to record the tension in the forehead muscles of his patients, he has been training them in deep muscle relaxation to fight the tension caused by stress. In an early study, six patients with elevated blood pressures achieved a drop of 11 percent, on the average, in both systolic and diastolic pressures. (Diastolic pressure occurs during expansion of the heart and systolic pressure during contraction of the heart as it beats.)

This particular technique is different from direct blood pressure feedback, and improvement takes a different course—no dramatic changes within a session, but an average decline over a period of instruction. What Dr. Love thinks is happening is that his patients are being taught to relax, with the result that there is less muscular pressure at the arteriole level—the small branches of the arteries. With less tension there may also be less energy fed into the hypothalamus, part of the brain that controls a number of internal functions.

What has any of this to do with pain? Everything. Avoidance of stress, learning to relax—these familiar terms have a direct effect on the tensions and learned behaviors which so often characterize chronic pain.

Electromyography or EMG, which records the changes in electric potential of muscle, appears to have the largest number of medical applications in this work, particularly for pain.

The voluntary or striated muscles are normally controlled by the individual out of the feedback he gets from his eyes, skin, and other sense organs. But there is no real feedback for muscle tension. He can be tense in a dozen areas without realizing it—in fact, over a period of years tension becomes habitual with him. It is here that EMG techniques are most helpful.

At the University of Colorado Medical Center, Dr. Thomas Budzynski and Dr. Johann Stoyva are working on tension headaches. With EMG leads attached to the patient's forehead, they monitor frontalis muscle tension and teach him to bring it down. Tension in these forehead muscles is a reliable indicator of general nervous tension. Also, says Dr. Budzynski, it is a good barometer of the emotions, even when the individual wears a poker face. "In our culture we learn to suppress exaggerated facial expressions. But I think residual EMG levels develop in certain muscles as a result of emotions, the frontalis among them."

If these frontalis muscles can be relaxed, the scalp, neck, and upper body muscles usually relax in turn. The Budzynski-Stoyva method has the patient in bed wearing earphones. The EMG leads on the forehead produce a tone in the headphones. The greater the muscle tension in the frontalis muscles, the higher rises the pitch in the headphones. The patient's task is to bring that pitch down. Early results indicate that it usually works.

At the Menninger Foundation in Topeka, Kansas, migraine headaches are being attacked with an entirely different type of biofeedback. This technique combines "temperature" biofeedback with "autogenic feedback training."

Autogenic training resembles autohypnosis in that it is a self-induced method of attaining inner calm and relaxation. It was first developed about 1910 in Germany by Johannes Schultz and has become popular in Europe. Autogenic feedback was discovered accidentally by psychologists Dr. Elmer Green, his associate E. Dale Walters of the Menninger Foundation, and Dr. Joseph E. Sargent, Chief of Internal Medicine.

Dr. Green had been using EEG, or electroencephalograph feedback, to control brain waves, with EMG (electromyography or muscle) feedback to reduce muscle temperature and increase the flow of blood in the patient's hands. The patient found that when she increased the temperature of her hands by ten degrees her migraine disappeared.

This experiment was duplicated successfully with a larger number of patients, some with migraine, some with tension headaches, and some with cluster migraine headaches. They worked with a temperature trainer that measured the difference in temperature between a forefinger and the forehead. They also studied a list of autogenic phrases: "I feel quiet," "My hands are warm and heavy," "My ankles, my knees, my hips feel heavy and relaxed."

The program, it is claimed, was so successful that within a month the patients did not need the feedback instrument. A year later the patients' progress was reviewed and improvement was judged at 74 percent, that is, 74 percent of the patients were significantly better.

The Menninger report says, "In our opinion, almost 100 percent of healthy persons have the physiological capacity to increase blood flow in the hands at will."

Dr. Seymour Diamond, Clinical Assistant Professor of Neurology at Chicago Medical School, whose work we have seen in the chapter on headaches, has also shown interest in biofeedback. *Medical World News* reports that he has treated (as of March 1973) some 200 patients with some variety of biofeedback technique.

Young patients, he says, respond best to temperature training if they are well motivated and if they have true migraine. It doesn't do much for people over thirty, or for those who have both migraine and depression headaches.

With EMG feedback, Dr. Diamond reports a 40 percent success rate compared with 25 percent using temperature training. He was skeptical at first of Budzynski's work, he says. "I was the first person to write about daily headaches as part of general depression, and I had treated a lot of such patients. After buying EMG equipment, I started to work with certain patients in whom everything else had failed. And about twenty intractable headache cases have responded admirably. These are people who have been through the mill. They don't respond to antidepressants; every other pharmacologic approach has been tried on them, and about half have had extensive psychotherapy as well, with no help."

Alpha wave feedback is still another method which appears to be of help in controlling pain. The EEG shows four patterns of human brain waves: alpha, beta, theta, and delta.

Briefly, beta waves have the highest frequency—14 or more cycles per second, and are associated with normal waking activity.

Down one rung are alpha waves, with 8 to 13 cycles per second, and characterized by a passive, relaxed, and tranquil state.

Theta waves are down another rung, with 4 to 7 cycles per second. The theta state is paradoxical, being associated with creative hallucinations or, occasionally, with anxiety.

Delta rhythms run from ½ to 6 cycles per second and are virtually always present in sleep.

Brain waves are only partially understood, but appear to be the result of the unceasing electrochemical activity in the cells of the brain. Like all nerve cells, brain cells transmit signals through a process of firing their energy along the fibers and this firing occurs in a synchronous pattern. The result is a rhythmic pulsing which can be detected at the surface of the scalp by an EEG machine.

The machine has three parts: a set of electrodes which are placed on the scalp to pick up the impulses, an amplifier to build the impulses up, and a panel of some sort to display them. Usually this comprises one or more pens tracing the patterns of firing on a moving roll of paper.

In our active waking states, beta waves do not occur in a smooth, regular flow, but in flurries of stop-and-go action, like bursts of static. By contrast, alpha waves are muted into a rhythmic tide which flows and ebbs over the cortex, usually from front to back. The significant factor is that the alpha state was discovered to be synonymous with calm, peace, and relaxation.

In 1958, Dr. Joe Kamiya was doing research in sleep at the University of Chicago and became fascinated by the alpha rhythms that he saw come and go in the EEG patterns. He began to wonder if people could be taught to be aware of the internal state these waves represented.

In his first experiment, a volunteer was set up in a darkened room with an EEG machine and told that a bell would ring at intervals, sometimes when he was in an alpha state, but sometimes when he was not. The question was: could he tell when the bell was right (for alpha) and when it was wrong?

The first day the subject was right about half the time—normal for the law of averages. The second day his score was 65 percent right; the third day 85 percent right. The fourth day he was 100 percent right, with 400 correct decisions made successively.

Eleven more subjects were able to repeat these results without any trouble.

How did they do it? They hadn't the faintest idea. More surprising yet, they were able to control their minds so completely that they could enter or leave the alpha state at will and sustain it as long as they wished.

In further experiments, Dr. Kamiya found that people could be taught to produce the alpha state in just a few hours. By modifying his equipment he produced a machine that would sound a note whenever alpha waves appeared. The subject had to learn to turn the note on and keep it on as long as possible. This turned out to be relatively easy to do.

The implications for pain control are striking. "This method," write Dr. Ronald Melzack and Dr. C. Richard Chapman, "appears to be effective for self-regulation of pain. Subjects are trained to increase the amount of alpha brain rhythm by providing a feedback signal (such as a tone) whenever alpha rhythm appears in their electroencephalogram. A high degree of alpha rhythm is associated with meditational states. The evidence so far is suggestive. Gannon and Sternbach reported that a subject who received alpha training was able to delay onset of migraine headaches by self-induction of the alpha state, but was unable to modify the pain after it was under way." [2]

Melzack and Chapman note four variables in biofeedback training that may give a boost to the job of beating pain.

One: distraction of attention. The patient switches his concentration from the painful site to the signal that is going on and off on the machine, and to the "inner-feeling" state that is being generated.

Two: the power of suggestion, the belief that what is happening is going to relieve the pain. In this respect, hypnosis can strongly potentiate the alpha training.

Three: the relaxation which accompanies the alpha state. Relaxation helps diminish pain by decreasing anxiety, turning off certain "arousal-provoking-inputs," and so on. Anxiety always sharpens the perception of pain, so decreasing anxiety tends to lessen the perception of pain.

[2] "Psychologic Aspects of Pain," *Postgraduate Medicine*, Vol. 53, No. 6, May 1973, pp. 69-75.

Four: development of a sense of control over pain. The idea that one is actually doing something about the pain promotes assurance, diminishes anxiety, and with it the pain. "The meaning of the pain differs depending on the presence or absence of control over it."

A program combining alpha training and hypnosis is being conducted by Dr. Melzack. The purpose of the hypnotic procedure, he says, is to teach the techniques of self-relaxation, to increase the motivation for asserting control over pain, and to create a state of greater receptivity to suggestion. Basically, the hypnosis is used to implant strong suggestions in the patient's mind that the alpha training will be successful. Which has the greater effect on the pain, the hypnosis or the alpha state, might be an interesting study in itself.

At the Seattle Pain Clinic, biofeedback attracted attention, says Dr. Roy Fowler, Jr., because of some of the problems in pain that seemed to be related to factors like muscle tension.

"We find that if we take these people who have been screened by physicians and they say they have muscle tension pains, and we put them in a machine that measures the EMG, the electrical output from the muscles, these people tend to produce higher amounts of electrical activity doing the same task that a normal person will do."

The tense muscle shows greater electrical activity. The patient testifies that it also produces pain. Does muscle tension produce the pain or does pain produce the muscle tension? Which came first, the chicken or the egg? It was this kind of question that intrigued Fowler and induced him to see if feedback could bring some answers where it could effect changes in the patient.

One of the questions that occurred to him was whether or not biofeedback was simply another form of hypnotism or suggestion.

"We do lots of things that lead you to suspect some connection. You've got flashing lights, and a doctor and his assistant who swoop down on the patient and pat him on the back when he does well, and show him graphs and say, 'Look, you're getting better,' and all these things must have an influence on him."

But there are as yet no good explanations for some of the procedures in biofeedback that seem to work. "We're in the interesting position of being able to see the behavior before we can really thoroughly explain it. Most of the work with biofeedback has outstripped the ability to explain the process. We know some of the critical elements that will make it effective. But if you ask me just exactly what happens when somebody changes his fingertip temperature, not only can't I tell you, but you can pick your own theory and we've got any number of physiologists working with us who will give you a good argument about it. There are people around the country who are devoting their whole professional lives to answering that question, or researching it.

"Here in Seattle, we're working primarily in two areas: muscle tension or muscle feedback. We are not only using our equipment to train people to reduce electrical activity or reduce muscle tension, but we are also training people who have problems like de-enervated muscles to increase electrical activity where it's appropriate. That means training somebody to use a muscle where it's partially de-enervated, or they're not getting a signal where they should be getting one.

"Now that's a learning process. You change the behavior in some way by giving the person information. And once you give him information he doesn't ordinarily have about some response, he can learn to control it. This is what we're doing with muscle and with temperature.

"One of my first studies was aimed at the question: how well do people perceive their muscle tension? They don't. They don't have any idea. The best correlation we got was almost perfectly backwards. Our subject said it was low when it was high and vice versa. So ordinarily we simply don't know what our muscles are doing—except at the extremes. You can tell when you are extremely tense. But with the aid of some really pretty simple electronic equipment you can measure this tension and then you can teach the person to begin to control it."

Dr. Fowler is working with temperature feedback on vascular headache, following the discoveries of Green and Sargent at the Menninger Foundation. But he is not wholly convinced there is a direct cause-and-effect relationship between increasing fingertip temperature and a relief of the migraine.

"We're researching it now. And we have a study design which I think will really answer some of these questions. In the meantime, however, I am forced to admit that training people to increase their fingertip temperature does seem to help them with their headaches. And it works with a high probability of success."

Dr. Fowler's goal at Seattle is to develop better techniques in biofeedback. "Techniques that can be used by the private practitioner in his office with equipment that is inexpensive and reliable, with procedures that are clear and can be replicated. I want to develop treatment approaches and treatment equipment and I would like very much to weed out some of these issues—how much of biofeedback is placebo, how much is suggestion, and how important is it to keep records and how much can you influence the therapy by altering the feedback you give to patients.

"One of the things we're testing now is the necessity of training people to perceive their tension. Just relaxing is fine, and we can do that. We can teach almost anybody to reduce his muscle tension dramatically. The real power of this feedback procedure is that just about anybody can learn it. And as far as we can tell, it works. It reduces pain. At least the patients claim it does. It's very difficult to measure pain."

In essence then, biofeedback consists of a group of techniques whose goal is to make available information otherwise not available; information about the state of brain waves, muscle tension, heartbeat rate, and so on. The revolutionary discovery involved in all this is that once this information is made available to the patient, he can learn to control involuntary functions of his body in a way that ordinarily would be completely beyond him.

If biofeedback can fulfill only part of its promise, the implications for controlling pain and improving individual health are remarkable.

Chapter 16

TERMINAL PAIN

Many people die of cancer without ever having any serious pain.
ROBERT G. PARKER, M.D.[*]

The patient lay quietly on his back, eyes nearly closed, his face slack from the effects of the narcotic. His voice was a hoarse, faint whisper.

"It starts out with an annoying, irritating little thing that you figure will be gone by night. And it goes on and it's worse—the next night it's worse. You go to your doctor to get some help and he tells you, 'Well, we'll do this or that,' and it seems to get a little better.

"Then, all of a sudden it breaks out in a different part of your body. And you begin to worry, you know? What's going on? So you go to a chiropractor and he does all kinds of different things to you and you feel pretty good and you go on your way and things seem to settle down.

"And then one day you find that you've got a cancer problem, but you have no pain at all, and what's he talking about? Cancer with no pain at all?

"So you go out and you start to check up on it, and all of a sudden you find that this thing is a freight train and somebody's

[*] Professor, Department of Radiology, University of Washington School of Medicine, Seattle, Washington.

pulled all the brakes loose on it, and it's running downhill at about 600 miles an hour.

"It attacks every joint, every bone, every blood vessel, every cell in your body, everything you're close to. It destroys them and one way or another you lose your body one part at a time.

"You begin to learn what pain is. You cannot any longer support the weight of your body. You cannot support the weight of your arms. You cannot talk. Someone has to raise your head up off the blanket so that you can move your jaw because the pain through the bone structure is so intense that you can't say anything but 'ouch.'

"It isn't continuous. There are times when you lie completely still and do nothing except think, 'I am not going to hurt.' Nothing happens. Then somebody walks into the room and says, 'Hey, have you seen last night's hospital paper?' And it all starts up again.

"The drugs we get today are very good. It would be nice if they would start quicker and last longer, and sometime between when they started quicker and lasted longer they would find a cure. The drugs make you sleepy all the time and tired, and you have no energy. . . ."

To most people this is cancer, though it is far from universally true. Says radiologist and cancer specialist Parker, "If you have a cancer clinic with a hundred patients, probably less than half have pain. Which is not meant to minimize it. The pain can be terrible, but it isn't true that all cancers produce major pain. Hodgkin's disease doesn't really cause pain unless it metastasizes or involves bone. Hodgkin's patients can go all the way through their illness with bizarre infections, blood problems and so forth, but may not have any pain. Fever is probably more important in Hodgkin's than pain. And leukemia—most patients, unless they have gingival infiltrates or bone involvement, may not hurt much.

"Cancer of the breast very often causes pain when it spreads to bone. That's a very common cause of it. On the other hand, if it just spreads on the chest wall, or sometimes involves the liver or the intestines or metastasizes to the brain it really doesn't cause a lot of pain. On the other hand, if it goes to the bone they really have it.

"Lung cancer—we have 45,000 men a year getting lung cancer

and they may not have pain, they may just suddenly bleed, which is mentally painful I suppose and frightening, but they may not hurt.

"The common concept of the terminal stages with excruciating pain—morphine and all that—well, it happens, but that is not the common way in which certain people have cancer. Cancer is so frequent a disease that even if a small complement has severe pain it's a big problem. And this is why the pain clinics get that sort of impression. Most people probably think that all or most cancer patients have pain because those are the ones we sent to the pain clinic."

Radiation treatment, says Dr. Parker, can effect real cures and it stops the pain. Heavy radiation can cause bone problems, but since this is local, it is a fair trade for a disease which was on its way to being fatal.

"When we treat cancer inside the oral cavity, particularly as it comes near the bone, and treat it for cure (which we can, many times), we have less than 3 or 4 percent incidence of problems with the bone itself. In the last ten years we probably haven't had more than five or six serious necroses of the bone.

"In those cases we may have cured the cancer but we've got the bone in trouble from the radiation. Now from our standpoint, when you're treating a lethal disease and you have only, say, a 1 percent incidence of severe complication, those are pretty good odds because you can get rid of the bone problem anyway.

"But then we send those people up to oral surgery and the only ones the oral surgeons see are the necroses and they think all our patients have necroses. They miss 99 percent of them."

Radiation damages bone by affecting the blood supply, narrowing the arteries, and killing the cells that form new bone.

"Most necroses can be treated conservatively if you can just get the mucosa to cover the dead bone. It really isn't bad unless it gets infected. It's not nice, but mouth cancer kills you. It's better to be alive and have a little problem—I think. But our oral surgeons must think we ruin bone in every patient. And if I worked in a pain clinic and saw all the cancer patients coming up there I'd think every patient must hurt.

"Medical students see the same thing with Hodgkin's. We had eight students here this summer and the only Hodgkin's patients they had ever seen were far advanced, with high fever. Then they walk in here and see a man with Hodgkin's who is on his way downtown to work in a law office and it astounds them. They thought everybody with Hodgkin's was up in the medical ward, dying. If we get Hodgkin's in a clinical stage one, we have a better than 80 percent survival rate. Not temporary either, they never have another problem with it."

Advanced cases are treated with combination drug therapy but the earlier stage—clinical stage one—can be halted with radiation.

"We use both cobalt and the linear accelerator. The accelerator is 8 million volts. Or we can use cesium, or neutrons."

The intense radiation shrinks solid tumor, and by shrinking it, relieves pain, for, if unhindered, the growing mass begins to invade other organs, blood vessels, and nerves. But the greatest cause of pain is when the cancer spreads to the bone. By this time the patient generally has already had surgery, so treatment of the bone is the next problem.

"If the spread is from breast cancer we can relieve better than 90 percent of those people's pain for the rest of their lives. Many of them have had the primary treatment years ago. We had one patient who had surgery thirty-two years before. Others come in with the pain and still haven't had the tumor diagnosed, like the one we saw this morning. We found it only on the mammography and it had already spread to the bone."

Another common impression which is not true is that breast cancer always spreads very fast—witness the patient with thirty-two years between the initial surgery and the later bone involvement. And even these long-standing conditions are still amenable to treatment.

"This patient will almost surely do well because she's already been able to win for thirty-two years and she'll probably win some more."

Where radiology is unable to check the pain, patients are sent to the pain clinic. The key to their operation is good communication between the pain clinic and the other specialties of the hospital so that each can play a decisive part in attacking the problem.

But where terminal pain is a problem, it must be faced, devastating as it can be to the patient, his family, even his physician.

"It is a problem," says Dr. Richard G. Black, coordinator of the

Seattle Pain Clinic, "because it is so very frequently mismanaged by physicians and mishandled by people themselves.

"Terminal pain is not only cancer. It can be other things— heart disease, liver disease—it's a condition with a hopeless prognosis.

"Let's consider what is done wrong in the average case. I was approached to help a lady because of a pain problem. I knew I could help her because her pain came from a cancer of the pancreas. The pain here is abdominal and we know, with this type of pain, that by doing alcohol nerve blocks on the nerves to the viscera (a relatively simple technique) we can render the person completely pain-free, with minimal side effects. This doesn't alter the course of the disease, you understand.

"We got a hurried consultation from the surgeon, rather young, very good, but without long experience in handling people. He wanted us to hurry up and block this patient so he could get her home by the weekend.

"It became apparent to us when we saw the patient the next morning that nobody had bothered to tell her what she had. And nobody had warned us about this.

"Someone, however, one of the relatives, had told the patient's son, who was having some teen-age problems of his own, and who somehow got the idea that his mother had only a week to live. Which was not correct either.

"We were met with hostility on the part of the patient who did not want to have anything to do with us because she didn't need any relief from her pain; she was going to get better anyway and the only thing that hurt her was her incision where she'd had her exploratory operation done and she was going to heal up and why should she see us?

"So we said, 'Fine,' and we didn't see any reason why she should either, and we left her. We went and had a talk with the surgeon who finally, under pressure, decided to break the news and tell her the truth.

"So they leveled with her and it took about two days to get things cleared around. We had their social worker and we have a nursing team that deals with terminally ill patients who come around and see the people and talk to the physicians first—sometimes they need more treatment than the patient.

"Once the patient knew the truth, she immediately took control of the situation. She calmed down, was no longer hysterical, told her husband that she was managing their money and he wasn't going to get one cent unless he stopped his damned drinking and straightened up before she died, and took charge of the son who had a minor drug problem—she really picked up 100 percent and became again an extremely rational person. She realized she was going to die and made very logical arrangements for it and behaved in the most unpredictable, calmest, businesslike fashion you'd ever want to see.

"We did the block on her, took away her pain, which ultimately relieved her of her medication, and gave her freedom from pain for at least six months. We explained carefully that this didn't affect the course of her disease. But if she later needed it, we could do other nerve blocks.

"Now two things happen when people die this way. First of all, they are pain-free and they don't have that terrible problem, with sleeplessness and the constant reminder of what is going on. Chronic pain, whether it be from arthritis, cancer, or anything else, is itself an exhausting thing for anybody—just complete physical exhaustion. And to be constantly reminded when you have a disease like this is also torment. That's one thing.

"The other thing is that when patients are relieved of their pain they don't need analgesics. And when they don't have analgesics, their heads aren't fuzzy, they think more logically, they don't panic. They are able to keep better control of themselves. We may even help this along by giving them mood-altering drugs at this time.

"With their minds clear they can be logical, we can reason with them, they can be with their families to the end, they can make whatever arrangements they want, they can enjoy their last days."

Enjoy? With death waiting? Dr. Black is totally realistic about it.

"Well, we all die. It's amazing, there have been many books written on death and dying and you get to realize it's an inexorable, logical process. Resentment first, and then acceptance— you go through all the stages.

"Now contrast this case," said Dr. Black, "with the death of a friend of mine, a physician. He was a gastroenterologist. He left Seattle to set up private practice in California. He'd had some gastrointestinal upset before leaving and got an upper GI series which the radiologist read as negative even though my friend thought there was a lesion there, but they called him a hypochondriac and talked him out of it.

"It became worse and finally he came to exploratory laparotomy and they found an advanced, inoperable cancer of the small bowel—a very rare tumor which he probably brought on himself by his research work, in which he had ingested some radioactive material about five years before.

"Now here's a young physician in his middle thirties, with a wife and two young daughters, seven and five, just getting started, and he's got less than a year to live.

"He was managed by a whole team of physicians. His wife, in her concern for him, became extremely manipulative about his management, phoning up one physician at eleven o'clock at night and then phoning up two others to confirm what the first one said, or playing one against the other. It was team management that didn't work out.

"All this came to me after the pattern had been established. One of the surgeons who knew what we were doing in the pain clinic got hold of me and said, 'You'd better get some help for Walter.'

"So I got Walter in and we did some nerve blocks on him and we rendered him pain-free. But Walter was never pain-free. By that time Walter was a drug addict. We attempted to withdraw him from the drugs but one of the physicians taking care of him took the attitude: well, he's going to die anyway. Let him have anything he wants. My attitude was the opposite. Don't give him any narcotics—we'll control his pain with other methods.

"Then somebody put in a hyperalimentation line, which meant that even though he was completely obstructed and his bowels weren't functioning, they were still continuing to feed him and keep him alive. It turned into a real horror story.

"They made arrangements for him to go home and he went through the phase of abandonment. There's no other way to describe it. One day there are seven doctors around you and the next day nothing. Or at least it must have seemed like nothing to him. There were only a few of us at the end.

"But from Walter's viewpoint, you're dying and you end up without any more appointments with a physician because every-

body has done everything they can do. And not through deliber-
ate action on anyone's part, but just because it works out that
you've exhausted all your appointments, you suddenly look at
your calendar one day, and you don't have any doctor to see.
Yet you're going to die and you don't quite know what to do, and
you feel completely alone and abandoned.

"And suddenly very frightened. No matter who you are. And
there was very little of the physician left in Walter at this time,
and there was one hell of a lot of narcotic left in him. We tried
several times to withdraw him with methadone and control his
medications, but there was interference between physicians and
there was his wife's attempt to do what she thought best—she
wanted him to die at home with his family around him—and he
ended up dying unnecessarily addicted.

"He died a miserable death at the wrong time—all the crying
and whining of a drug addict every couple of hours for a fix. He
was no longer a human being; he was as much an addict as somebody on the street, scared and demanding—and there was nothing to be done with him. He wanted the drug and he knew how
to get it.

"So, contrasting these two—there are miserable ways to die
and better ways to die, but I think in our society there's no excuse for dying a drug addict. Because narcotics do not relieve
pain for a prolonged period of time. They are good for short-term
pain relief, then they go. And if they are used for long-term pain
relief, they have to be used in a very, very special way, on a
time-contingency basis, and without the ups and downs that you
get with short-acting narcotics.

"The other way to die is with a group of people who appreciate—psychologically and psychiatrically—the problems of dying,
are willing to support the person at the appropriate time, and
who can render him pain-free by techniques other than narcotics: nerve blocks, cordotomies, that sort of thing.

"Of course we're limited by what nerve blocks we can do in
the dying patient by the side effects of the block. We don't want
to paralyze anyone unnecessarily, make them lose control of
their sphincters, bowels, or bladders, because this is often more
disabling than the disease at the time. In these areas a neurosurgical intervention is probably better.

"When the pain is in the trunk, or about the head and neck,
we are quite capable of handling blocks even at early stages.

But if it involves a limb, an extremity, we prefer not to do a block but rather a more definitive neurosurgical procedure. There you have more control and fewer side effects. Sometimes a nerve block is a shotgun approach, while with neurosurgery you can be more discreet, like picking out the parts you want with a rifle. Or, you can go central and do something like a cordotomy that interferes with central pain pathways rather than peripheral nerve blocks.

"Early in my career I made a few mistakes. I had a man with lung cancer that was eating into his chest wall and who was in agonizing pain in spite of a heavy narcotic program. I took away all his pain very simply in one little procedure by putting alcohol in his spinal cord and blocking all the pain coming in from his trunk.

"The next thing I knew, I had a man who was wide awake, who knew he was going to die and had not been psychologically prepared for it. He was no longer sedated with medications—his physician had simply stopped all his drugs because he didn't have any more pain. You can't do that, you have to taper off gradually.

"So we ended up with a raving maniac who needed drugs because of his addiction and who knew he was going to die and had absolutely no sedation for it or psychological preparation for it.

"The whole thing is in the team approach. Part of it is the relief of pain and the other part is getting the patient to realize and accept the inevitability of what is going to happen.

"We learn the hard way sometimes, but we learn. One reason we learn is that we are looking for feedback. We follow up, we want to know what happens to people and to their families. This is essential if you're going to learn anything from the whole experience.

"For instance there was Walter, my physician friend. We have 150 or more hours of videotape on his last days. He did a lot of it himself and everybody who took care of him did it and it takes in everyone—his family and the minister and everyone involved. This has all been abstracted into a short course on death and dying.

"It's something I've got strong feelings about because it's done wrong so often—not through malice but, I think, through a sense of utter futility on the part of most physicians who have never anywhere in their medical training been prepared for this, or even know what is available to them for help.

"So what does the average physician do? He gets out of it somehow. You use your natural escape mechanisms and you get out of it. Either you give the person narcotics so they shut up and go away, or you let someone else take care of them—the hospital. You do as the nurses do, you put them in a back room and try to forget about them. Because every time you see them you are reminded of your own helplessness.

"And you shouldn't be, because I think this is the place you can be most helpful. You try to fight the attitude that says, 'You can't do anything for him. Give him all the drug he wants.' All you have to do sometimes is to take a few days off or a weekend, and you come back and it's done. The patient is back on narcotics, or sent home on narcotics, or something like that.

"It takes a lot out of you. But something has to be done for these patients. There's no funding for this kind of program. You can get money for cancer research, but you can't get money to help people die. It takes a lot of money. By the time the chronic pain patient comes to us in the pain clinic, it's the end of a long road. He's seen lots of doctors. He has spent, or had spent on him, hundreds of thousands of dollars. That's what has been removed from our economy. His earning power has been destroyed, his family has to be supported, the medical bills have to be met. And it adds up to a psychologically and economically devastating experience for any family."

In the face of this devastation, Dr. Black insists, it is piling on still another burden to allow the patient to become addicted to narcotics and then watch him deteriorate to something less than human. Relief from pain, yes, but not with addictive drugs, not when there are techniques like nerve block which will bring relief, in most cases, without the destruction of personality resulting from drugs. It is all the more important in the case of terminal pain, when the temptation is strong to let the patient have anything he wants, to spare him and those caring for him those final dreadful moments.

It takes a very special kind of human being to face this kind of horror every day, to retain his sanity and perspective, to continue to do whatever he possibly can to banish pain, to help, in however large or small a measure, to the best of his ability.

Chapter 17

DENTAL PAIN

As the use of anesthetic agents of any kind in the extraction of teeth is attended with inconvenience, nearly always delaying the operation, the author is of the opinion that their employment, as a general thing, should be dispensed with.

CHAPIN A. HARRIS [1]

Do you sometimes harbor the unhealthy suspicion that your dentist is at worst a sadist or at best indifferent to your pain? The heavy hand on the drill, the bland disregard of those drops of perspiration on your suffering brow, seem to indicate a certain lack of sensitivity. After all, why are you wincing like that? You got a shot of novocaine, didn't you? Hold still and open wider.

That injection of novocaine you got was a nerve block in the real sense of the word. Properly placed, it does a good enough job of producing local analgesia. Yet, apparently, it is not enough, for 60 percent of the American populace avoid the dentist on any and every pretext and thousands more really go into a panic at the prospect of a session in the chair. As for the miraculous shot of novocaine which will take away all the pain, dentists themselves say that patients seem to fear the needle most of all, regarding it with a special kind of horror.

[1] *The Principles and Practice of Dentistry,* 11th edn., revised by F. J. S. Gorgas, P. Blakiston Son & Co., Philadelphia, Pa., 1885.

There are dentists, fortunately, who are not merely mechanical marvels, who are humane and compassionate, and who have devoted a great deal of their lives to finding new methods for controlling pain.

Recognized throughout the world is the Loma Linda technique taught at the School of Dentistry of Loma Linda University in California and for more than fifty years associated with the name of Niels Bjorn Jorgensen, D.D.S.*

Professor Jorgensen, born in Denmark, practicing and teaching in California, recognized early that fear, anxiety, and apprehension compounded the patient's distress and magnified his pain. If these factors could be reduced, he thought, the anesthetic would work much more effectively. Over five decades he has experimented with and studied various combinations of drugs for this purpose.

Reduced to its simplest terms the technique taught by Professor Jorgensen at Loma Linda combines preliminary sedation with the following analgesic. He administers one or another of several sedatives or tranquilizers before the pain-killer to calm the patient's anxiety and help control the apprehension or fear. It has been found also that the sedative may boost by synergistic action the effect of the local anesthetic used.

This same principle is now widely employed in general surgery where the patient is sedated before going up to the operating room where he receives the anesthetic.

Perhaps this doesn't sound like a revolutionary idea, but it was a breakthrough even as late as the mid-forties when Dr. Jorgensen's work began really to be recognized. And even today, not so many dentists will take the extra time and trouble required for this careful preparation of the patient.

Dr. Jorgensen's techniques are very precise. The first step is a complete medical history of the patient, with detailed questions about any existing disease conditions such as diabetes, angina pectoris, high blood pressure, or coronary thrombosis. He checks blood pressure and pulse, and in the case of any cardiovascular condition will make additional checks such as a breath-holding test to determine the patient's functional reserve. If the

* Emeritus Professor of Oral Surgery, School of Dentistry, Loma Linda University, Loma Linda, California.

patient cannot hold a full breath for more than fifteen seconds, he is regarded with considerable medical suspicion.

The good dentist tries also to make a psychological evaluation of his patient. He considers the problems of fear and anxiety and balances them against the personality type as he judges it. Does the patient show any signs of being paranoid, compulsive, hysterical, or schizoid? Any such tendency affects their relationship and the treatment.

The hysterical personality gags easily and has a low tolerance for fingers or instruments in his mouth. On the credit side, he is suggestible and easily influenced and responds to a firm, reassuring manner.

The compulsive personality is a rigid perfectionist, and nothing is ever done quite satisfactorily for him. The new inlay is out of line, the bite isn't right, there's a rough edge—the adjustments can go on endlessly.

The paranoid personality is suspicious and distrustful. He is defensive and irritable and questions procedures the normal patient would readily accept. He requires much more explanation to disarm his suspicions.

The schizoid personality is aloof and cold, maintains a wall of reserve between himself and the dentist, and stiffens at any form of personal contact. These patients require much more tact, patience, and understanding than they usually get from a busy practitioner, many of whom work on two or even three patients simultaneously.

The oral personality is one whose major preoccupations revolve around activities of his mouth—eating, drinking, chewing, or smoking. His reaction to the dentist may be one of complaints, with demands for more attention than normal or essential, and with irritability and quick changes of mood.

Obviously the dentist is faced with numerous situations in which the patient will tolerate pain poorly, react unpredictably, and, often enough, pose emotional and psychological problems. Extreme cases, of course, cannot be treated, but within manageable bounds the use of simple psychotherapeutic measures combined with premedication are invaluable.

Such short-term and improvised psychotherapy needs to be simple and supportive, consisting of reassurance, a calm, friendly, warm, and confident attitude. Anticipating anxiety or fear and taking steps to reduce it are important. Above all, the dentist needs to take the time to win the patient's confidence. To do this he must be willing to explain in detail exactly what he intends to do. One of the greatest sources of anxiety to the apprehensive patient is the mysterious and formidable preparations going on around him which he does not understand and which appear to portend the most gruesome results. A full explanation, so that he knows what is going to be done and why, is invaluable.

Also helpful is letting the patient talk, letting him bring out some of his fears—about pain, about loss of teeth, and so on. That way his questions can be satisfied and reassurance offered. This simple psychotherapy is groundwork for the sedation and anesthesia to follow.

Sedation is not given routinely to every patient. There is no need to give sedatives or narcotics for a short and simple operation. But for the bigger job it can make quite a difference.

"For lengthy procedures of restorative dentistry, the patient should be spared the simple stress imposed by the grinding and manipulation. Sedation is a 'must' for any prolonged or severe oral surgery, such as multiple extractions involving any difficulty, or the removal of impacted teeth with the patient under local anesthesia." [2]

Sedation does not mean unconsciousness. The dental patient is ambulatory and the goal is to keep him ambulatory, not to knock him out with heavy drug dosage. Therefore sedation is administered with a light hand, unlike the procedure in a hospital for surgery where it doesn't matter how sleepy he gets.

If light sedation or tranquilization is all you need, couldn't you, on your way to the dentist, simply pop a tranquilizer first so that you would arrive relaxed and unafraid? Dr. Jorgensen says no. Tranquilizers were tried for this purpose but, in his opinion, are not wholly satisfactory. When combined with barbiturates or narcotic analgesics, they can lead to a sudden depression of the respiratory center or an unpleasant drop in blood pressure. Moreover, when the patient takes it upon himself to do the premedication, the intake is not precisely controlled, and

[2] Niels Bjorn Jorgensen and Jess Hayden, Jr., *Sedation: Local and General Anesthesia in Dentistry,* [various contrib.] Lea & Febiger, Philadelphia, Pa., 1972, p. 21.

like most medical people, Dr. Jorgensen frowns on this kind of self-administered shotgun therapy. "In our experience," he says, "neither the oral nor the intramuscular route has proven as effective as intravenous sedation of patients."

Finally, the choice of the sedative is important. The ideal drug would just depress some of the higher brain centers, bypassing the medula which controls the vital autonomic functions such as respiration and blood circulation. It would act quickly and fade quickly, leaving no hangover. Such a drug has yet to be discovered. There are, however, a number of available chemicals which are very useful.

Closest to the ideal, in Dr. Jorgensen's opinion, is a combination of nitrous oxide (laughing gas) and oxygen. Nitrous oxide in large doses is an anesthetic itself, but he does not use it in that way. Mixed with 50 percent or more of oxygen, it provides light sedation, complete relaxation, relief from fear and apprehension, and induces a pleasant mood. The patient is fully conscious and cooperative. Once the work is finished, a few minutes of oxygen washes out the remaining nitrous oxide and eliminates any possibility of hangover.

Employed this way, nitrous oxide appears to have a very high safety factor. In Denmark, where it is used much more widely than in the United States, four million treatments were given between 1956 and 1970 without a single case of serious complications.

Three patients under treatment were observed one morning in Dr. Jorgensen's private practice in Los Angeles and exhibited closely similar attitudes. Mr. A, a television actor, took his place in the chair without hesitation or anxiety, and had the nosepiece adjusted.

According to Dr. Jorgensen's method, the air vent on the nosepiece is closed and the bag is filled with oxygen alone, with the flowmeter set at ten liters a minute, a flow rate suggested by Dr. Gerald Allen and Dr. Gaither Everett of the University of Washington. The patient breathes oxygen for two minutes, then the flow of nitrous oxide is begun at the rate of one liter a minute and the oxygen is reduced by one liter a minute. After that the nitrous oxide is increased one-half liter a minute, while the oxygen is decreased one-half liter a minute, keeping the total gas minute-volume constant, until a base line is reached. At this base

line the patient describes his sensations as being pleasantly relaxed, with occasional tingling in hands and lips.

Dr. Jorgensen asks the patient to keep him continually informed as to his feeling of relaxation. He is also instructed that
he can control his level of sensation by asking for more or less of
the nitrous oxide or simply by taking in room air through his
mouth.

Mr. A reported that he felt completely relaxed; he was slightly
dizzy, but that it was a wholly pleasant feeling. He regarded the
approach of the needle with serenity and was given an injection
for the lower jaw (inferior alveolar nerve block) which goes into
the gum tissues behind the lower molars.

Dr. Jorgensen injected the novocaine with extreme slowness,
taking several minutes to complete the injection. Thereafter,
grinding and fitting of a restoration proceeded without the
slightest sign of strain to the patient. When his mouth was mo-
mentarily free of instruments or fingers, he carried on a normal,
pleasant conversation about Hollywood and the television industry. When the session was finished, he left the chair without
the usual attitude of relief that the ordeal was over—it had
obviously not been an ordeal for him.

The second and third patients observed that morning displayed
the same cheerful attitude and indifference to stress, while describing the same sensations.

If for some reason the patient objects to the gas or the mask
over his nose, there are alternatives. Nearly as good as nitrous
oxide are some of the short-acting barbiturates such as secobarbital (Seconal) or pentobarbital (Nembutal).

Pentobarbital is sedative in small doses, hypnotic in larger
doses, and anesthetic in still larger doses. Assuming only sedation
is desired, pentobarbital can be given orally fifteen to twenty
minutes before operation as the simplest procedure, but Dr.
Jorgensen dislikes the oral route because he finds results less
dependable. They are apt to vary at different times, even with
the same patient, being affected by the contents of the stomach.
Other observers have pointed out that results are affected merely
by the time of day, the so-called circadian rhythm of our bodies.

Dosage is determined by the patient's age, weight, and tem-
perament, but if his tolerance is unknown it is started at one half
the average hypnotic dose. If this is not effective, it is repeated

in half an hour. The aim is not to pass beyond sedation into hypnosis, for this corresponds to general anesthesia which poses its own problems.

For Dr. Jorgensen, the intravenous method, in which the drug is slowly injected into a vein, has clear advantages. "By injecting the drug *very slowly* the dentist can obtain almost immediately an index of the patient's individual reaction to it, and the desired degree of sedation can be established. Although the intravenous route is generally considered to be the most dangerous of all, if employed with optimum care it possibly is one of the safest." [3]

In what is a fairly traumatic experience for the patient, like having a tooth extracted, he might combine pentobarbital with meperidine (Demerol) and scopolamine. Demerol is a strong analgesic of the morphine class (see Chapter 8), but it also has some sedative value. Given together with a barbiturate it appears to boost the action of the barbiturate, raises the pain threshold, and gives the patient a sense of well-being.

Its disadvantages are that it is a narcotic and cannot be given frequently without some risk of addiction. It also depresses the respiration centers and the heart. It should never be given to patients who are taking mood-elevating drugs of the MAO class such as isocarboxazid (Marplan). Last and not least, Demerol can stimulate the vomiting center and cause the patient to gag and retch.

As early as 1940, Dr. Jorgensen experimented with pentobarbital to control gagging. He was giving it by mouth then, and he found it did counteract the nausea produced by Demerol. In one difficult case, a thirty-five-year-old man who gagged every time a finger or instrument was put in his mouth, it took six grains of pentobarbital taken orally to control the spasms.

Seven years later, when new work needed to be done, Dr. Jorgensen gave sodium pentobarbital intravenously. Less than 100 mg. of the drug, or somewhere between one quarter and one third as much as the oral dose, was needed to achieve the same result. Dr. Jorgensen found this ratio to hold with other difficult patients as well. The 100 mg. dose is somewhat higher than that needed for ordinary sedation.

[3] Jorgensen and Hayden, *Sedation: Local and General Anesthesia in Dentistry*, p. 25.

It seems certain that pentobarbital, in addition to its sedative effect, does depress the gagging center. "For that reason," he said, "it occurred to me that it might also be used before meperidine is administered." [4] He then worked out a method of administering pentobarbital intravenously with $\frac{1}{300}$ to $\frac{1}{200}$ grain of scopolamine added, followed by 25 to 50 mg. of meperidine. This combination effectively controlled nausea and gagging.

Scopolamine is a good sedative and tranquilizer, and can be useful in another way—it reduces the flow of saliva, which is obviously desirable during the time the patient's mouth is full of instruments and fingers. Atropine sulfate is used in similar fashion.

Finally, in the roster of useful drugs, there are the numerous tranquilizers. Some mentioned in dental literature are diazepam (Valium), promethazine (Phenergan), and hydroxyzine (Atarax or Vistaril). The authoritative British handbook *SAAD* refers to Atarax as "enjoying increased popularity with anaesthesiologists and dentists. Rapid-acting and mild, hydroxyzine exhibits sedative and tranquilizing powers along with antihistaminic properties." [5]

Dr. Jorgensen considers Valium also worth a trial for clinical procedures which do not last longer than forty-five minutes. It produces muscular relaxation, anticonvulsant action, promotes calm, and induces some amnesia. There are undoubtedly patients for whom this would be a real benefit—they would like to forget the whole thing once it is over.

On the whole he still prefers the nitrous oxide/oxygen combination, or the short-acting barbiturates. Valium needs care in use; he feels it should not be used for elderly patients who may be confused, for patients with glaucoma, for those taking barbiturates, MAO inhibitors, or alcohol. And he does not like the feeling of euphoria which persists for many patients as long as eight hours after a 10 mg. dose. This effect, according to *SAAD*, can be one, not merely carefree, but of "sheer irresponsibility."

[4] "Control of Nausea from Meperidine (Demerol)," *Southern California State Dental Association Journal*, Vol. 23, April 1955, pp. 32-33.
[5] Robert B. Steiner, "Drug Intoxication," *Intravenous Anesthesia SAAD*, 5th edn., ed. S.L. Drummond-Jackson, Society for the Advancement of Anaesthesia in Dentistry, London, 1971, p. 376.

In establishing a condition of light sedation with barbiturates, a base line is reached similar to the procedure with nitrous oxide. Pentobarbital is injected very slowly while the patient is carefully watched for the first sign, which may be drowsiness, dizziness, or a slight blurring of vision. This is the base line. It may require anywhere from 30 mg. to 300 mg. of the barbiturate to reach this point.

Once the base line is reached, a small additional quantity of pentobarbital is added, about 10 percent more. The aim is not to go beyond light sedation. Then the Demerol is added. The dentist should have resuscitative equipment on hand—oxygen and a pressor drug such as phenylephrine to counteract a sudden drop in blood pressure.

In England, a barbiturate called methohexitone is popular for short dental procedures. It is known in the United States as methohexital, trade-named Brevital. The 1971 edition of *SAAD* says that in ten years of use in Britain there has not been a single death due to this drug. Brevital is used as an intravenous anesthetic alone or in combination with other agents for a more prolonged anesthesia, but Dr. Jorgensen considers it best used for operations lasting no longer than twenty minutes.

Another barbiturate, sodium thiopental (Pentothal) is also widely used in the United States for short operations, although Brevital appears to be the drug of choice for ambulatory patients because it has a shorter action and so allows accurate control of the depth of anesthesia by small intermittent doses. Still, say two prominent oral surgeons, both methohexital and thiopental "provide a rapid, excitement-free induction and also have the advantage of an amnesic effect which permits many non-painful procedures to be done when the patient is apparently awake. Therefore, no unpleasant postoperative memory ensues." [6]

The majority of patients seem to find their experience with Brevital a pleasant one. Their perception of time is affected and the session in the dental chair appears shortened. The effect then wears off rapidly and patients are usually able to walk away

---

[6] Adrian O. Hubbell and R. Quentin Royer, "A Method of Outpatient General Anesthesia for the Oral Surgical Patient," from *Sedation: Local and General Anesthesia in Dentistry*, by Jorgensen and Hayden et al, Lea & Febiger, Philadelphia, Pa., 1972, pp. 91-101.

without trouble after a short rest. There are occasional after-effects—weeping for a few minutes during the recovery period is not uncommon according to Hubbell and Royer, but it is over in ten or fifteen minutes and is later not even remembered by the patient. Sometimes anxiety with wringing of the hands, sleeplessness, and crying may occur, and this may last twenty-four hours or more. Pentobarbital taken orally after the patient returns home is effective for this condition.

Brevital can be combined with nitrous oxide to smooth out the action and prevent an up-and-down pattern of anesthesia depth. The patient who remains restless under Brevital alone can be given a small additional dose of Valium (5 mg.) or Demerol, which some practitioners consider the drug of choice.

Painless dentistry has been a promise ever since the early perambulating operators who used half a bottle of whiskey as their anesthetic. With the development of novocaine, and then lidocaine and mepivacaine it came a great deal closer. And with wider adoption of such scrupulous techniques using premedication, fear of the dentist may yet be reduced to the vanishing point.

The Loma Linda technique was a breakthrough in pain control. Dr. Jorgensen continues to teach at Loma Linda and his original discoveries have been picked up and amplified by others doing new pioneer work in their own fields, such men as Jess Hayden, Jr., Professor and Associate Dean of the College of Dentistry at the University of Iowa, Adrian Hubbell of Long Beach, California, who studied with Dr. Lundy at the Mayo Clinic and advanced the knowledge of intravenous anesthesia, and two men from the National Institutes of Health in Bethesda, Maryland, both with a broad understanding of the public health aspects of pain control in dentistry: Edward J. Driscoll, Chief of the Anesthesiology Section, and Aaron Ganz, Chief of the General Oral Sciences Program.

There are many others working in this vital area of pain control, fitting together another piece of the jigsaw puzzle that comes closer bit by bit to rounding out the picture. We still only half understand pain, but the work of these men and others like them have brought this much enlightenment: it isn't necessary to hurt if you know what to do about it.

Chapter 18

WHAT YOU CAN DO

This is not a how-to-do-it book, but unavoidably one amasses a liberal collection of dos and don'ts. Sprinkled throughout these pages have been caveats of many kinds. The informed patient, demanding more detailed explanations, may be trying to a busy doctor, but he is better able to deal with his own problems. To deal with problems it is necessary to admit they exist. It is therefore vital to recognize the warning signs, as described by Dr. Richard G. Black of the Seattle Pain Clinic.

The first major sign, to be underlined in red, is: If you are using a short-acting analgesic, something you take every two or three hours, and you have been taking it for more than a week (two weeks at most) and still have pain, something is wrong—especially if you've increased the dose or the frequency.

Your next step is to recognize or admit what has happened to you since you have had this pain. Has it diminished your ability to function effectively, to do your job, keep house, or enjoy a normal social life and recreational activities? If so, in what way has it interfered? Are other people doing your job for you? Are you leaning on friends or colleagues, using pain as an excuse not to function?

Another warning comes out of your relationships with other people, especially your family. Are you more irritable? Are there more conflicts and more fights? Is there more tension around the house between yourself and your children or your spouse? Has your sex life suffered? Is the situation continuing to deteriorate?

If you see these warning signs, you'd better get help.

Let's construct a hypothetical situation which may be encountered almost daily at a pain clinic.

You become aware that your back has been hurting a little too frequently. When you lift something there's pain, and sometimes if you even sit a little crooked in a chair it hurts. At the dinner table, if you reach for something, sometimes there's pain.

You think back to that time last summer when you fell out of the boat and hurt yourself. That was three or four months ago; funny it should be hurting now. But it is, and it seems to have gotten worse.

You try to ignore it, but it doesn't go away. So finally you decide you'd better do something about it. Inside, you're worried. You don't really want to see a doctor for fear of what you may find out. You keep telling yourself that you don't want to act like a hypochondriac and run to the doctor for every little ache, after all, it isn't really that bad.

But finally you do go. Your wife has noticed your wincing every now and then and has begun to nag you to see a doctor, and it's time for a routine checkup anyway. You tell the doctor about this pain in your back. He listens to your story and he examines you. He says he doesn't see anything wrong and tells you to use a heating pad.

So you go home and for a week you try heat, but the pain doesn't change. You phone the doctor and tell him there's been no change. He says he'll call the drugstore and give them a prescription for you and asks you to phone him in a week.

You try these pills all week long but nothing sensational happens, so you go back to the doctor and he reexamines you and arranges to have some X-rays taken of your back. Later, he calls you to say that nothing showed up on the X-rays and advises, "Stay on the medication for awhile."

You continue taking the medication and somehow the weeks slip by and you realize the pain is still there and it's bothering you more than ever. It's not that the pain is actually worse, but you are more conscious of it. You can't get the thought of pain out of your mind and you are getting very tired of it. It drags you down and, whether it is or is not more severe, it seems worse.

You've had several different prescriptions filled by now and perhaps have even tried cortisone injections, but nothing has helped. You're becoming depressed. You realize that these trips to your doctor are expensive and not very productive. He goes through much the same routine each time and reassures you, but you realize he's not really doing very much for you. So you ask him, "Shouldn't I see someone else about this? We're not getting anywhere."

Your doctor might be just about to suggest this himself, but, being human, when *you* say it, he appears a little stung. The tone of his voice tells you he is annoyed. "Oh, I don't think we need to do that. I think we can handle this all right." Or, on the other hand, perhaps he graciously says, "Yes, of course. I think we should." And he refers you to a specialist.

You see the specialist and, after some tests, he recommends that you go into the hospital for a day for more studies. After this there's a consultation with your doctor and the specialist. They suggest that if the pain is really becoming that much of a burden to you, they would recommend surgery. You agree, hoping for a complete, almost magical, cure.

If you are lucky, surgery, or any of the other things done, solves the pain problem and the story ends here. But in some cases it doesn't.

If you are one of these cases, you go on. You've seen three doctors, had one operation, been given a lot of medication, and you still have the pain. Your depression is worse. You're beginning to wonder if these doctors know their business. Your wife may say they are stupid, your friends can describe a hundred cases of faulty diagnosis where people who were treated for one condition turned out to have something else entirely. You are getting a lot of annoying flak from your associates and you are still taking a lot of medicine.

The pain has now assumed a more important place than ever in your life. It may in fact be no more severe than when you first debated about going to the doctor, but your whole attention is presently focused on it and it is in the driver's seat, running your life.

You've begun to lose confidence in your doctors. You may even have tried going to a chiropractor or an acupuncturist. Yet, if you assess the situation carefully, you will find that in all this time—

several months, perhaps—you have had only brief periods with your doctors. And only during these few brief periods have you actually talked about your pain problem or emphasized how badly it is affecting your life. The rest of the time you've kept it to yourself, concealed it from your spouse so as not to worry her (or him) about it. You've tried to minimize it to yourself, yes, even to the doctor. To begin to think of it as serious is frightening. Maybe there's a little machismo in you—you don't want to seem less than the stalwart male. You shrink from the cry-baby image if you are a woman, so you refuse to become tragic about it and worry your husband. You try to hide it from him.

The doctor doesn't realize how badly this is affecting you and he's never had a conversation with your spouse about how it is altering your family life. Everybody who comes to him comes with a complaint and it is normal for him to hear complaints all day. You haven't gotten through to him with the real measure of this pain and how it is affecting you. He may still assume it is relatively minor. Apparently, you're still able to function, you haven't lost your job or outworn the patience of your spouse.

Of course you have come back several times with complaints, but then so do a lot of his other patients. And a lot of them complain incessantly about things he knows to be minor, so there is always that possibility you want to avoid—being tagged by him as a complainer.

Where do you go from here? Now is the time to do these things:

1. Sit down and make a list of the doctors you have seen and describe briefly what each has done. List them chronologically.
2. Make a second list of the medications you have taken. Have your wife or husband check both lists.
3. With your spouse or a friend, go to your medicine cabinet and take out all the bottles with your name on them that you are not actually taking now. Throw them away. All this medication is dangerous to have in the house and may be a crutch to your illness.

If you do this, and study your lists conscientiously, several things should become apparent. The principle revelation may be to prove to you just how serious the problem actually is.

If you have now seen seven or eight doctors, have had roughly fifteen different medications, and are taking more than one pill a day, you are in trouble. We are talking, of course, about pain. There are other conditions for which you may be taking medication on a long-term basis—some stomach medicine, digitalis for the heart, or something of that nature.

Now you can see the shape of the problem. You have too many doctors, have taken too much medicine, and are not getting better. The time has come to face it. You are a chronic pain patient.

Your next move is back to the doctor. But which one among the many you have seen?

Dr. A is kind and considerate. You know that if you complain about the pain, he will give you a prescription. A small voice whispers to you that you can always manipulate Dr. A into giving you a prescription. But, in the light of your newly compiled lists, is that good?

Dr. B is very busy. Going to see him may mean a long wait in a crowded office run by a harried nurse or assistant. But when you finally do get in to see Dr. B, he doesn't rush you. He spends a lot of time with you, and you feel pretty good after talking to him. Not until later do you realize that he hasn't done very much for you. He won't give you much in the way of medication and says aspirin is enough.

Dr. C is reserved, almost cold, very efficient. Right in the middle of your story he interrupts you. "We've got to get some tests done. I want you to check into the hospital next Wednesday. We'll get some more X-rays and run some additional tests. I'll phone you after we get the results. Goodbye."

So you put your emotions aside and pick Dr. C. You go to the hospital for the tests. Suddenly you are in a dehumanized world where nobody explains anything to you except to say "Stand here" or "Stand there." Mechanized robots do frightening things and there seems to be nothing human on the other end at all.

You go home and, after a few days, you get a call from the nurse to come in to see Dr. C. He has your X-rays and tests and he tells you in his crisp, efficient way that you need an operation. Can you be ready by Thursday?

It may not happen just this way. This is a composite picture and probably a little extreme, but it isn't unreasonable. It can and does happen in much this way. Remember that you come to the doctor demanding help. It puts him in the kind of spot where he must do something for you, and so this chain of events occurs often enough.

But what are your alternatives? Suppose that instead of Dr. A, B, or C, you went to Dr. D, who is in group practice? For your first interview you meet a physician who spends some time talking to you because that is his job. He is the *triage* physician (the French term for "sorting") who assesses the patient's problems and decides whether he should see the orthopedic specialist, the internist, the psychiatrist, or what should be done in general.

This is a departure from the individual, private practice of medicine. Under ordinary circumstances, the *patient himself* unknowingly makes the largest part of the decision as to what will be done merely by the doctor he selects.

For example, if the patient with acute appendicitis goes to *any* physician, he will end up having an operation for it. That's the optimum procedure. If he has a mild coronary and goes to any physician, he will probably end up with the usual treatment—morphine, bed rest, and the other traditional things.

But if he has something more obscure, something in a gray area, the situation changes. If he selects a surgeon, he will get what the surgeon has to offer: surgery. If he selects an internist, he will get what the internist has to offer: medicine. If he selects a psychiatrist, he will get what the psychiatrist has to offer: psychotherapy. It is unfortunate that this choice can be made unknowingly by the patient, as it so often is. This is why so many specialists operate on a referral basis. The route should be through a general practitioner—family medicine specialist is the new term—who will take care of minor problems and send you on to a specialist if more help is needed.

Another possibility is the special clinic that offers a full medical work-up. This corresponds in a way to Dr. D's approach. The special clinic can be a little warmer than the dehumanized laboratory described above because it has interns, residents, and nurses who can talk to the patients and provide some human touch. The big question is whether or not the work-up is appropriate to the problem.

Teaching hospitals provide good care with more supervision. Their residents, who are very good, quite conscientious, and well-motivated, are supervised by specialists.

What the specialists provide the residents with, in addition to close supervision, is back-up experience. Reciprocally, the residents offer the specialists the latest basic knowledge out of the medical schools. The combination in a teaching hospital is a very good one.

The patient's first responsibility to himself is to face up to his problem and to document it with his lists or with a diary. His second task is to break down the communication barrier between himself and his doctor, to present the physician with evidence of how serious the problem has become for him, and to stress the need for doing something about it without appearing to be a crank.

If he compiles a list of doctors he has seen and medications he has taken, keeps some sort of diary of what has been going on (without being overly compulsive about it), and tells the physician what is happening inside him, he is then in a position to ask for more help. He can ask his doctor to refer him to a larger medical center, like a university hospital, which usually attracts specialists of high caliber.

If the patient gets no satisfaction from his doctor, he has the right to end his relationship with this physician. But if he does so, he should end the relationship formally, not just disappear and go to another doctor. For one thing, it puts the new doctor in the position of taking a patient away from a colleague, which can embarrass him and damage the relationship right at the start. But more important, the new physician needs the patient's medical records from the first doctor. There is much more information in these medical records than in the patient's incomplete version of the many procedures he has been through. The transfer of these records from one doctor to the next is the essential key to the changeover.

The structure of our medical system is such that it assumes a one-to-one relationship between doctor and patient. It assumes that patients are not accumulating several doctors working in ignorance of each other's existence. This one-to-one relationship is invaluable for establishing personal contact with feelings of confidence and trust. But under some conditions it may be an obstacle between the patient's requirements and his ability to get additional help. The one-to-one relationship is both the strength and the weakness of the system. It is not yet clear what

202 The Conquest of Pain

the ultimate solution may be, for the antithesis of the one-to-one system is group medicine, which has its own problems.

In the meantime, the patient should seek the immediate goal of having himself admitted to a larger medical center, perhaps a pain clinic, by referral from his doctor.

This book cannot recommend pain clinics. Only the patient's physician can do this. There are a variety of pain clinics, many of which have not been covered in our discussions. Some are one-man clinics and some are special-purpose clinics, like those devoted to acupuncture, where a single approach to every problem is offered. In the opinion of experts cited in this book, the multidisciplinary clinic is to be preferred. There are still comparatively few of these and the only route to one is through your own doctor.

He will either know of such a clinic or he can find out where one is through his medical society or through the American Medical Association. In any case, you, the patient, could not walk into a pain clinic, if you knew of one, and have yourself admitted. As in a hospital, admission can only be arranged by a physician. If you do have an intractable pain problem, this is your route.

In the end, the patient's problem is that of finding a good doctor and the physician's problem is in being a good doctor. The old-fashioned family physician knew the people in his community inside out. He cared for their ills, delivered their babies, and knew pretty much everything about them. He knew whose father was an alcoholic, whose child was adopted, and who was in trouble. He knew the community so thoroughly that, if you just gave him your address, he could tell you how you grew up and what childhood diseases you'd had. In big, impersonal cities the doctor no longer knows all these details about the people and the community, the intimacies of their lives that affect their responses to illness and health.

On the other hand, yesterday's doctor didn't have the techniques and the drugs that are now available. He couldn't do the things for his patients that can now be done. But mushrooming technology has brought its own problems. One physician cannot now master the whole technology of medicine as he once did, any more than he can know all about the personal lives of his patients in our crowded, complex society.

Since he cannot know all the technology, he must be free to

call in additional technical help in the medical specialties when it appears to be necessary. He should also feel free to get help from the paramedical specialties—the psychologists, the social workers, and others—to round out his treatment of the individual patient.

Therein lies the key to the multidisciplinary clinic: the goal of treating the whole man, the whole family unit. This is now difficult for the individual physician to do. The patient sees a doctor who, more often than not, is overworked, staggering under a crushing case load. For the most part, the doctor simply does not have the time to listen patiently to what is being said, analyze an endless story of symptoms, and then make the decision that this may or may not be the real problem, that there may be something else underlying these symptoms which the patient is not able to express, describe, or even understand himself. His real problem may be loneliness, fear, depression, inadequacy, sex—a hundred possibilities he cannot bring himself to discuss frankly with a man who is still a stranger to him. But with a deeper insight into the nature of his problem, he is in a better position to help his doctor help him.

We have come a long way since the first witch doctors and faith healers tried to banish pain with bell, book, and candle. There is still some distance to go.

Appendix

The first International Symposium on Pain was held in Seattle, Washington, May 21–26, 1973, with Dr. John J. Bonica as chairman. The conference was sponsored jointly by the University of Washington School of Medicine and the National Institutes of Health, with added financial support by a number of business organizations.

Participants and speakers came from a dozen countries and totaled 102 in all, primarily research-oriented physicians and specialists in the physiology and psychology of pain. The full text of the papers delivered are now available as part of the "Advances In Neurology" series, Volume 4, published by Raven Press, 15 West 84th Street, New York, N.Y. 10024.

For those interested in particular aspects of pain research, the agenda, in abbreviated form, follows. Note: Asterisked entries indicate that the speaker's credentials and affiliations have been previously given.

A. RECENT INVESTIGATIONS

PERIPHERAL MECHANISMS

Receptors and Spinal Nerves

"Activation of Cutaneous Nociceptors and Their Actions on Dorsal Horn Neurons," A. Iggo.
AINSLEY IGGO, D.SC., PH.D., Professor, Department of Physiology,

Faculty of Veterinary Medicine, University of Edinburgh, Edinburgh, Scotland.

"Patterns of Discharge Evoked in Cutaneous Nerves and Their Significance for Sensation," P. R. Burgess.

PAUL R. BURGESS, PH.D., Associate Professor of Physiology, University of Utah College of Medicine, Salt Lake City, Utah.

"Activity in Unmyelinated Nerve Fibers in Man," Rolf G., Hallin and H. Erik Torebjörk.

ROLF HALLIN, M.D., Department of Clinical Neurophysiology, Academic Hospital, Uppsala, Sweden.

"Total Afferent Inflow and Dorsal Horn Activity upon Radiant Heat Stimulation to the Cat's Footpad," Manfred Zimmermann and Hermann O. Handwerker.

MANFRED ZIMMERMANN, Physiologishes Institut, Universität Heidelberg, Germany.

Discussion

Biochemical Aspects

"Biochemical Mechanism of Ischemic Pain," F. Sicuteri, G. Franchi, and S. Michalacci.

FEDERIGO SICUTERI, M.D., Professor and Chairman of Clinical Pharmacology and Director of the Headache Center, University of Florence, Florence, Italy.

"Pain—A General Chemical Explanation," Olov Lindahl.

OLOV LINDAHL, M.D., PH.D., Professor of Orthopedics, Orthopedic Center, Regionsjukhuset, Linkoping, Sweden.

Discussion

Cranial Nerves

"Electron Microscopy of Deafferentation in the Spinal Trigeminal Nucleus," Lesnick E. Westrum.

LESNICK E. WESTRUM, M.D., PH.D., Assistant Professor, Departments of Neurological Surgery and Biological Structure, University of Washington School of Medicine, Seattle, Washington.

"Responses of Facial Cutaneous Thermosensitive and Mechanosensitive Afferent Fibers in the Monkey to Noxious Heat Stimulation," R. Dubner, R. Sumino, and S. Starkman.

RONALD DUBNER, D.D.S., PH.D., Chief, Neural Mechanisms Section, National Institute of Dental Research, National Institutes of Health, Bethesda, Maryland.

"An Evaluation of Duality in the Trigeminal Afferent System," Lawrence Kruger and James A. Mosso.
LAWRENCE KRUGER, PH.D., Professor of Anatomy, UCLA Center for Health Sciences, Los Angeles, California.
"Identification of Central Trigeminal Nociceptors," Luke M. Kitahata, Roseanne G. McAllister, and Arthur Taub.
LUKE M. KITAHATA, M.D., PH.D., Associate Professor of Anesthesiology, Departments of Anesthesiology and Neurosurgery, Yale University School of Medicine, New Haven, Connecticut.

Discussion

Sympathetic Nervous System

"Pain and Autonomic Nervous System," D. Gross.
DIETER GROSS, M.D., Facharzt für innere Medizin und Nervenkrankheiten, Arbeitskreis für neurovegetative Therapie, Krankenhaus Maingau vom Roten Kreuz, Frankfurt/Main, Germany.

Discussion

Pain Threshold

"Studies on the Pain Threshold in Man," P. Procacci, M. Zoppi, M. Maresca, and S. Romano.
PAOLO PROCACCI, M.D., Associate Professor of Medicine and Director of Pain Center, University of Florence, Florence, Italy.
"An Alternative to Threshold Assessment in the Study of Human Pain," C. Richard Chapman.
C. RICHARD CHAPMAN, PH.D., Research Assistant Professor, Departments of Anesthesiology and Psychology and Anesthesia Research center; Member, Pain Clinic, University of Washington School of Medicine and College of Arts and Sciences, Seattle, Washington.

Discussion

CENTRAL MECHANISMS

Ascending Pathways in Spinal Cord

"Central Pain and the Spinothalamic Tract," William R. Mehler.
WILLIAM R. MEHLER, PH.D., Associate Professor of Anatomy (Adjunct), University of California Medical Center, San Francisco, California, Neurosciences Branch, NASA-Ames Research Center, Moffett Field, California.
"The Primate Spinothalamic Tract as Demonstrated by Anterolateral

Cordotomy and Commissural Myelotomy," Frederick W. L. Kerr and Harry H. Lippman.

FREDERICK W. L. KERR, M.D., Professor of Neurosurgery, Associate Professor of Neuroanatomy, Mayo Graduate School of Medicine, Rochester, Minnesota.

"Origin of Spinothalamic and Spinoreticular Pathways in Cats and Monkeys," D. Albe-Fessard, A. Levante, and Y. Lamour.

DENISE ALBE-FESSARD, D.Sc., Professor, Physiologie Nerveuse, University of Paris VI, Paris, France.

"Location and Functional Properties of Spinothalamic Cells in the Monkey," Daniel L. Trevino, Joe D. Coulter, R. A. Maunz, and William D. Willis.

DANIEL L. TREVINO, Department of Physiology, School of Medicine, University of North Carolina.

"Relationships Between Activity in Spinal Sensory Pathways and 'Pain Mechanisms' in Spinal Cord and Brainstem," Irving H. Wagman and James A. McMillan.

IRVING H. WAGMAN, PH.D., Professor of Physiology, School of Medicine, University of California, Davis, California.

"Modulation of Dorsal Horn Throughput by Anesthetics," James E. Heavner and Rudolph H. de Jong.

JAMES E. HEAVNER, D.V.M., PH.D., Assistant Professor, Department of Anesthesiology, University of Washington School of Medicine, Seattle, Washington.

Discussion

Brainstem

"The Midbrain and Pain," B. S. Nashold, Jr., W. P. Wilson, and G. Slaughter.

BLAINE S. NASHOLD, JR., M.D., Associate Professor of Neurosurgery, Duke Medical Center, Durham, North Carolina.

"Bulboreticular and Medial Thalamic Unit Activity in Relation to Aversive Behavior and Pain," Kenneth L. Casey, James J. Keene, and Thomas Morrow.

KENNETH L. CASEY, M.D., Associate Professor of Physiology, University of Michigan Medical School, Ann Arbor, Michigan.

"Effects of Bradykinin Intra-Arterial Injection into the Limbs upon Bulbar and Reticular Unit Activity," J. M. Besson, G. Guilbaud, and M. C. Lombard.

JEAN-MARIE BESSON, PH.D., Chemist, Laboratoire de Physiologie des Centres Nerveux, Paris, France.

Discussion

Brain

"Thalamic Convergence and Divergence of Information Generated by Noxious Stimulation," David Bowsher.

DAVID BOWSHER, M.A., M.D., PH.D., Reader in Neurobiology, Department of Anatomy, The University of Liverpool, Liverpool, England.

"Cortical Representation of Aδ Tooth Pulp Primary Afferents in the Cat," L. Vyklicky and O. Keller.

LADISLAV VYKLICKY, M.D., D.SC., Institute of Physiology, Czechoslovak Academy of Sciences, Prague, Czechoslovakia.

Discussion

Descending Control Systems

"On the Induction of Prolonged Change in the Functional State of the Spinal Cord," V. C. Abrahams.

VIVIAN C. ABRAHAMS, PH.D., Professor of Physiology, Queen's University, Kingston, Ontario, Canada.

"Descending and Segmental Control of C Fiber Input to the Spinal Cord," A. G. Brown, W. C. Hamann, and H. F. Martin III.

ALAN G. BROWN, B.SC., M.B., CH.B., PH.D., Research Fellow, Department of Veterinary Physiology, University of Edinburgh, Edinburgh, Scotland.

"Central Mechanisms of Pain Inhibition: Studies of Analgesia from Focal Brain Stimulation," John C. Liebeskind, David J. Mayer, and Huda Akil.

JOHN C. LIEBESKIND, PH.D., Associate Professor of Psychology, University of California School of Medicine, Los Angeles, California.

Discussion

Psychologic Aspects

"Psychological Concepts and Methods for the Control of Pain," Ronald Melzack.

RONALD MELZACK, PH.D., Professor of Psychology, McGill University, Montreal, Quebec, Canada.

"Measuring the Severity of Clinical Pain," Richard A. Sternbach, Robert W. Murphy, Gretchen Timmermans, Jerry H. Greenhoot, and Wayne H. Akeson.

RICHARD A. STERNBACH, PH.D., Adjunct Associate Professor of Psychiatry, School of Medicine, University of California San Diego, La Jolla, California.

"The Placebo Response in Pain Reduction," Frederick J. Evans.
FREDERICK J. EVANS, PH.D., Associate Professor of Psychology in Psychiatry; Senior Research Psychologist, Unit for Experimental Psychiatry, Institute of the Pennsylvania Hospital and University of Pennsylvania, Philadelphia, Pennsylvania.

Discussion

PAIN RESEARCH: CURRENT STATUS AND FUTURE OBJECTIVES

"The Future of Attacks on Pain," Patrick D. Wall.
PATRICK D. WALL, M.A., D.M., Professor of Anatomy; Director, Cerebral Functions Research Group, University College, London, England.

PATHOLOGIC ASPECTS

Peripheral Nerve Disorders

"Observations on the Treatment of Denervation Dysesthesia with Psychotropic Drugs: Postherpetic Neuralgia, Anesthesia Dolorosa, Peripheral Neuropathy," Arthur Taub and W. F. Collins, Jr.
ARTHUR TAUB, M.D., PH.D., Associate Professor of Neurology and Neurophysiology (Surgery), Yale University School of Medicine, New Haven, Connecticut.

Discussion

Phantom Limb Pain

"Central Neural Mechanisms in Phantom Limb Pain," Ronald Melzack.*

"Relief of Phantom Limb Pain: A new Operative Method," Olov Lindahl.*

Discussion

Central Pain States

"Pathologic Aspects of Central Pain States," W. Noordenbos.
W. NOORDENBOS, M.D., PH.D., Professor of Neurosurgery, University of Amsterdam, Amsterdam, The Netherlands.

"Pain Due to Central Nervous System Lesions: Physiopathological Considerations and Therapeutical Implications," Carlo A. Pagni.
CARLO A. PAGNI, M.D., Associate Professor of Neurosurgery, University of Milan, Milan, Italy.

Discussion

Pathophysiology of Oral Pain

"Responses of Stomatognathic Structures to Noxious Stimuli," Yojiro Kawamura.
YOJIRO KAWAMURA, M.D., D.M.Ss., Professor and Head, Department of Oral Physiology, Dental School, Osaka University, Osaka, Japan.
"Electrical Stimulation of Human Teeth and Convergence in the Trigeminal System," J. M. Mumford and A. V. Newton.
J. M. MUMFORD, PHD., M.Sc., M.S., F.D.S.R.C.S., Senior Lecturer in Operative Dental Surgery, University of Liverpool; Consultant Dental Surgeon, United Liverpool Hospitals, Liverpool, England.

Discussion

Visceral Pain

"Problems of Visceral Pain," Chuji Kimura, Kengo Tsunekawa, Kaoru Kumada, and Kenjiro Mori.
CHUJI KIMURA, M.D., Professor of Second Surgical Department, Kyoto University Medical School, Kyoto, Japan.
"Heart Pain," P. L. Del Bianco, E. Del Bene, and F. Sicuteri.
P. L. DEL BIANCO, University of Florence, Florence, Italy.

Headache

"The Serotonin (5-HT) Theory of Migraine," F. Sicuteri, B. Anselmi, and M. Fanciullacci. °
"Vascular Permeability and Vasoactive Substances: Their Relationship to Migraine," Donald J. Dalessio.
DONALD J. DALESSIO, M.D., Professor of Neurology; Associate Dean for Clinical Affairs, University of Kentucky College of Medicine, Lexington, Kentucky.
"Recent Observations on Migraine, with Particular Reference to Thermography and Electroencephalography," Arnold P. Friedman, A. James Rowan, and E. H. Wood.
ARNOLD P. FRIEDMAN, M.D., Clinical Professor of Neurology, Co-

lumbia University College of Physicians and Surgeons; Physician-in-Charge, Headache Unit, Montefiore Hospital, Bronx, New York. [Retired]

Discussion

Chronic Pain Behavior

"Pain Viewed as Learned Behavior," Wilbert E. Fordyce.
WILBERT E. FORDYCE, PH.D., Professor of Psychology, Department of Rehabilitation Medicine; Member, Pain Clinic, University of Washington School of Medicine, Seattle, Washington.
"Varieties of Pain Games," Richard A. Sternbach.*

Discussion

B. DIAGNOSIS AND THERAPY

GENERAL DIAGNOSTIC AND THERAPEUTIC METHODS

"Organization and Function of a Pain Clinic," John J. Bonica.
JOHN J. BONICA, M.D., Professor and Chairman, Department of Anesthesiology and Anesthesia Research Center; Director, Pain Clinic, University of Washington School of Medicine, Seattle, Washington.

Diagnostic and Therapeutic Nerve Blocks

"Current Role of Nerve Blocks in Diagnosis and Therapy of Pain," John J. Bonica.*
"Diagnostic and Therapeutic Nerve Blocks: Recent Advances in Techniques," A. P. Winnie, S. Ramamurthy, and Z. Durrani.
ALON P. WINNIE, M.D., Professor and Head, Department of Anesthesiology, Abraham Lincoln School of Medicine, University of Illinois Hospitals, Chicago Illinois.

Discussion

"New Local Anesthetics for Pain Therapy," Benjamin G. Covino.
BENJAMIN G. COVINO, PH.D., M.D., Scientific Director, Research and Development Division, Astra Pharmaceutical Products, Inc.;

Lecturer, University of Massachusetts School of Medicine, Worcester, Massachusetts.

"Current Role of Neurolytic Agents," Jordan Katz.
JORDAN KATZ, M.D., Professor and Associate Chairman, Department of Anesthesiology, University of Wisconsin School of Medicine, Madison, Wisconsin.

"Subarachnoid Saline Perfusion," V. Ventafridda and R. Spreafico.
VITTORIO VENTAFRIDDA, M.D., Professor and Head, Pain Department, National Cancer Institute of Milan, Milan, Italy.

"Treatment of Post-Traumatic Sympathetic Dystrophy," Harold Carron and Robin M. Weller.
HAROLD CARRON, Department of Anesthesiology, University of Virginia Medical Center, Charlottesville, Virginia.

Biophysical Methods

"Selective Use of Radiation Therapy for the Cancer Patient with Pain," Robert G. Parker.
ROBERT G. PARKER, M.D., Professor, Department of Radiology, University of Washington School of Medicine, Seattle, Washington.

"The Role of Physical Medicine in Problems of Pain," Barbara J. DeLateur.
BARBARA J. DELATEUR, M.D., M.S., Associate Professor, Department of Rehabilitation Medicine; Member, Pain Clinic, University of Washington School of Medicine, Seattle, Washington.

Discussion

Nonaddictive Analgesics

"Studies on Mechanisms Underlying Non-Narcotic Analgesia," Jeffery L. Barker and Herbert Levitan.
JEFFERY LANGE BARKER, M.D., Special Fellow, National Institute of Neurological Diseases and Stroke, Behavioral Biology Branch, National Institute of Child Health and Human Development, National Institutes of Health, Bethesda, Maryland.

"Recent Advances in Non-Narcotic Analgesics," Abraham Sunshine.
ABRAHAM SUNSHINE, M.D., Associate of Clinical Medicine, New York University Medical Center; Attending Physician, Knickerbocker Hospital, New York, New York.

Discussion

Narcotics

"Are Synthetic Narcotics Adequate Substitutes for Opium-Derived Alkaloids?" William T. Beaver.

WILLIAM T. BEAVER, M.D., Associate Professor of Pharmacology and Anesthesiology, Georgetown University Schools of Medicine and Dentistry, Washington, D.C.

"The Use and Misuse of Narcotics in the Treatment of Chronic Pain," Raymond W. Houde.

RAYMOND W. HOUDE, M.D., Associate Professor, Departments of Medicine and Pharmacology, Cornell University Medical College; Attending Physician, Memorial Sloan Kettering Cancer Center, New York, New York.

Discussion

Other Drugs

"Psychotropic Drugs and the Management of Chronic Pain," Lawrence M. Halpern.

LAWRENCE M. HALPERN, PH.D., Associate Professor, Department of Pharmacology; Member, Pain Clinic, University of Washington School of Medicine, Seattle, Washington.

"The Mechanisms of Action of Anti-Inflammatory Agents in the Control of Pain," Robert F. Willkens.

ROBERT F. WILLKENS, M.D., Clinical Associate Professor of Medicine, University of Washington School of Medicine, Seattle, Washington.

Discussion

Other Methods of Therapy

"Treatment of Pain by Changing the Acid-Base Balance," Olov Lindahl.*

PSYCHOLOGIC AND PSYCHIATRIC METHODS

Hypnosis

"Pain Suppression by Hypnosis and Related Phenomena," Martin T. Orne.

MARTIN T. ORNE, M.D., PH.D., Professor of Psychiatry; Director of

Unit for Experimental Psychiatry, Institute of the Pennsylvania
Hospital and University of Pennsylvania, Philadelphia, Pennsylvania.
"Clinical Use of Hypnosis in Pain Management," Basil Finer.
BASIL FINER, M.B.B.S., M.D., F.F.A.R.C.S., D.A., Associate Pro-
fessor in Anaesthesiology and Intensive Care, University of Uppsala,
Uppsala, Sweden.

Discussion

Operant Conditioning

"Treating Chronic Pain by Contingency Management," Wilbert E.
Fordyce.°

Discussion

Psychologic and Psychiatric Methods

"Conjoint Treatment of Chronic Pain," Jerry H. Greenhoot and Richard
A. Sternbach.
JERRY H. GREENHOOT, M.D., Assistant Professor of Neurosurgery,
School of Medicine, University of California San Diego, Veterans
Administration Hospital, San Diego, California.
"The Contribution of the Psychiatrist to the Treatment of Pain,"
H. Merskey,
HAROLD MERSKEY, D.M., M.R.C. Psych., Physician in Psychological
Medicine, The National Hospital for Nervous Diseases, London,
England.

Discussion

NEUROSURGICAL ABLATIVE TECHNIQUES

Dorsal Rhizotomy

"Dorsal Rhizotomy: Indications and Results," John D. Loeser.
JOHN D. LOESER, M.D., Assistant Professor, Department of Neuro-
logical Surgery; Member, Pain Clinic, University of Washington
School of Medicine, Seattle, Washington.
"Rhizotomy: What Is Its Place in the Treatment of Pain?" Burton M.
Onofrio.
BURTON M. ONOFRIO, M.D., Assistant Professor of Neurological
Surgery, Mayo Graduate School of Medicine, University of Minne-
sota, Rochester, Minnesota.

Discussion

Sympathectomy

"Sympathectomy for the Relief of Pain," James C. White.
JAMES C. WHITE, M.D., Professor of Surgery (Emeritus), Harvard Medical School and Massachusetts General Hospital, Boston, Massachusetts.

Discussion

Mechanisms and Treatment of Cranial Neuralgias

"Postsynaptic Repetitive Neuron Discharge in Neuralgic Pain," B. L. Crue and E. J. A. Carregal.
BENJAMIN L. CRUE, M.D., Chairman, Division of Clinical Neurology; Director, Department of Neurosurgery, City of Hope National Medical Center, Duarte, California.
"A Laboratory Model for Trigeminal Neuralgia," Richard G. Black.
RICHARD G. BLACK, M.D., Assistant Professor, Department of Anesthesiology and Anesthesia Research Center; Coordinator, Pain Clinic, University Hospital, University of Washington School of Medicine, Seattle, Washington.
"Interaction of Noxious and Non-Noxious Stimuli in Primary Sensory Nuclei," Robert B. King.
ROBERT B. KING, M.D., Professor and Chairman, Department of Neurosurgery, State University of New York, Upstate Medical Center, Syracuse, New York.
"Controlled Thermocoagulation of Trigeminal Ganglion and Rootlets for Differential Destruction of Pain Fibers: 1. Trigeminal Neuralgia," William H. Sweet and J. G. Wepsic.
WILLIAM H. SWEET, M.D., D.Sc., Professor of Surgery, Harvard Medical School; Chief, Neurosurgical Service, Massachusetts General Hospital, Boston, Massachusetts.

Discussion

Percutaneous Cordotomy

"Percutaneous Cordotomy (R.F.)," John F. Mullan.
JOHN F. MULLAN, M.D., M.B., B.CH., B.A.O., John Harper Seeley Professor and Head, Section of Neurosurgery; Director, Brain Research Institute, University of Chicago Hospital and Clinics, Chicago, Illinois.
"Percutaneous Radiofrequency Cervical Cordotomy for Intractable Pain," Hubert L. Rosomoff.

HUBERT L. ROSOMOFF, M.D., Professor and Chairman, Department of Neurological Surgery, University of Miami School of Medicine, Miami, Florida.

"A Stereotactic Approach to the Anterior Percutaneous Electrical Cordotomy," S. Lipton, E. Dervin, and O. B. Heywood.

SAMPSON LIPTON, M.B., CH.B., F.F.A.R.C.S., Director, The Centre for Pain Relief, Department of Medical and Surgical Neurology, The Walton Hospital, Liverpool, England.

Discussion

Other Techniques

"Place of Stereotactic Technique in Surgery for Pain," Carlo A. Pagni.*

"Chemical Hypophysectomy for Cancer Pain," Guido Moricca.

GUIDO MORICCA, M.D., Professor of Anesthesiology and Director of Pain Center, National Cancer Institute Regina Elena, Rome, Italy.

"The Suppression of Pain by Intrathalamic Lidocaine," Vernon H. Mark and Hiroshi Tsutsumi.

VERNON H. MARK, M.D., Associate Professor of Surgery, Harvard Medical School; Director, Neurological Surgery, Boston City Hospital, Boston, Massachusetts.

Discussion

NEUROSURGICAL STIMULATION TECHNIQUES

Transcutaneous and Peripheral Nerve Stimulation

"Percutaneous Local Electrical Analgesia; Peripheral Mechanisms," Arthur Taub and James N. Campbell.*

"Conduction Failure in Thin Nerve Fiber Structures and Accompanying Hypalgesia During Repetitive Electric Skin Stimulation," H. E. Torebjörk and R. G. Hallin.

ERIK TOREBJÖRK, M.D., Department of Clinical Neurophysiology, Academic Hospital, Uppsala, Sweden.

"Stimulation of Pain Suppressor Mechanisms: A Critique of Some Current Methods," William H. Sweet and J. G. Wepsic.*

"Peripheral Nerve and Cutaneous Electrohypalgesia," Howard L. Fields, John E. Adams, and Yoshio Hosobuchi.

HOWARD L. FIELDS, M.D., PH.D., Instructor in Neurology and Physiology, University of California Medical Center, San Francisco, California.

"Cutaneous Afferent Stimulation in the Treatment of Chronic Pain,"
Donlin M. Long and Margaret Tuohy Carolan.
DONLIN M. LONG, M.D., PH.D., Associate Professor of Neurological
Surgery, University of Minnesota Hospitals, Minneapolis, Minnesota;
(Professor Designate, Neurological Surgery, Johns Hopkins University, Baltimore, Maryland).
"Acute Pain Control by Electrostimulation: A Preliminary Report,"
Alan C. Hymes, D. E. Raab, E. G. Yonehiro, G. D. Nelson, and
A. L. Printy.
ALAN C. HYMES, M.D., Thoracic and Cardiovascular Surgeon, St.
Louis Park Medical Center; Clinical Assistant Professor of Surgery,
University of Minnesota School of Medicine, Minneapolis, Minnesota.

Dorsal Column Stimulation

"Physiological Effects of Dorsal Column Stimulation," H. Friedman,
B. S. Nashold, Jr., and G. Somjen.
H. FRIEDMAN, Memphis Neurological Clinic, Memphis, Tennessee.
"Six Years' Experience with Electrical Stimulation for Control of Pain,"
C. Norman Shealy.
C. NORMAN SHEALY, M.D., Director, The Pain Rehabilitation Center, S.C., La Crosse, Wisconsin.

Thalamic Stimulation

"Chronic Thalamic and Internal Capsular Stimulation for the Control
of Facial Anesthesia Dolorosa and Dyesthesia of Thalamic Syndome," Yoshio Hosobuchi, J. E. Adams, and H. L. Fields.
YOSHIO HOSOBUCHI, M.D., Assistant Professor, Department of Neurological Surgery, University of California Medical Center, San Francisco, California.

Discussion

ACUPUNCTURE

"Effects of Acupuncture Stimulation on Activity of Single Thalamic
Neurons in the Cat," Mark Linzer and Loche Van Atta.
MARK LINZER, B.S., Senior Scholar, Department of Chemistry,
Oberlin College, Oberlin, Ohio.
"Acupuncture for Chronic Pain in Japan," Toru Sato and Yoshio
Nakatani.

Toru Sato, M.D., Professor and Chairman, Department of Anesthesiology, Tottori University School of Medicine, Yonago, Japan.

"Pain, Acupuncture, Hypnosis," Ronald L. Katz, C. Y. Kao, Herbert Spiegel, and Gail J. Katz.

Ronald L. Katz, M.D., Professor of Anesthesiology, Columbia University College of Physicians and Surgeons, New York, New York; (Professor and Chairman Designate, Department of Anesthesiology, UCLA Medical Center, Los Angeles, California).

"Acupuncture and Experimentally Induced Ischemic Pain," Gene M. Smith, Han T. Chiang, Richard J. Kitz, and Alia Antoon.

Gene M. Smith, Ph.D., Departments of Anesthesiology and Pharmacology, Massachusetts General Hospital, Boston, Massachusetts.

Discussion

Index

Masochism, 28, 111
Melzack, Ronald, 13–19, 22, 23, 24, 26, 27, 171, 172
Melzack-Wall gate theory of pain, 13–19, 22, 91, 150, 151, 161
Meperidine, 74, 191, 192
Mepivacaine, 194
Mesmer, Franz, 38–39
Methadone, 68, 69, 75–76
Methohexital, 193
Methohexitone, 193
Methysergide maleate, 134
Migraine, 124–125, 127, 131
 biofeedback technique and, 168
 causes of attacks, 133
 classic, 130
 cluster, 130
 common, 129
 drug treatment for, 134, 136–137
 See also Headaches
Miller, Neal E., 166
Milton, John, quoted, xi
Miracles, 47, 48
Moncey, George, 48
Morphine, 66–67, 74–75, 77, 84, 139, 152
Morrison, James D., 83 *fn.*
Müller, Johannes, 11
Mystics, 45

N

National Institute of Mental Health, 69
National Institute of Neurological Diseases and Blindness, Committee on Classification of Headache, 127
Nembutal, 190
Nerve blocks, 8–9, 26, 52–53, 55, 69, 85–88, 182–183, 184, 185

Nerve fibers, pain and, 10–11
Neural pain, 8
Neurectomy, 89
Neurosurgery, 85–92
Nitrous oxide, 189–190, 192, 194
Nobel, Alfred, 125
Noise, white, use to distract patient's attention, 22, 90–91
Nonorganic pain, 2–3
Norpramin, 135
Novocaine, 185, 190, 194
Nupercaine, 87

O

Operant conditioning, 93–107, 113, 140
Opiates, 65–69
Organic pain, 3
Orne, Martin T., 138–139
Oxycodone, 74
Oxyphenbutazone, 72

P

Pain
 kinds of, 7–9
 learned, 8–9
 nature of, 5–9
 neurophysiology of, 55
 new approach to, 1–4
 protracted, 9
 psychogenic, 21, 33, 95, 108
 psychology of, 20–34, 56
 referred, 7–8
 tension, 26
 terminal, 175–184
 theories of, 18–19
 therapy of, 2
Pain (journal), xiii